CAMBRIDGE LIBRARY COLLECTION

Books of enduring scholarly value

History of Medicine

It is sobering to realise that as recently as the year in which On the Origin of Species was published, learned opinion was that diseases such as typhus and cholera were spread by a 'miasma', and suggestions that doctors should wash their hands before examining patients were greeted with mockery by the profession. The Cambridge Library Collection reissues milestone publications in the history of Western medicine as well as studies of other medical traditions. Its coverage ranges from Galen on anatomical procedures to Florence Nightingale's common-sense advice to nurses, and includes early research into genetics and mental health, colonial reports on tropical diseases, documents on public health and military medicine, and publications on spa culture and medicinal plants.

The Works, Literary, Moral, and Medical, of Thomas Percival, M.D.

A physician and medical reformer enthused by the scientific and cultural progress of the Enlightenment as it took hold in Britain, Thomas Percival (1740–1804) wrote on many topics, including public health and demography. His influential publication on medical ethics is considered the first modern formulation. In 1807, his son Edward published this four-volume collection of his father's diverse work. Some of the items here had never been published before, including a selection of Percival's private correspondence and a biographical account written by Edward. Volume 4 contains the third and fourth parts of Percival's *Essays Medical and Experimental*, which were completed following the revised edition that is reissued separately in one volume in the Cambridge Library Collection. The essays reflect Percival's wide range of interests, such as the regulation of hospitals and prisons, and the medical abnormalities he sometimes observed in his patients.

Cambridge University Press has long been a pioneer in the reissuing of out-of-print titles from its own backlist, producing digital reprints of books that are still sought after by scholars and students but could not be reprinted economically using traditional technology. The Cambridge Library Collection extends this activity to a wider range of books which are still of importance to researchers and professionals, either for the source material they contain, or as landmarks in the history of their academic discipline.

Drawing from the world-renowned collections in the Cambridge University Library and other partner libraries, and guided by the advice of experts in each subject area, Cambridge University Press is using state-of-the-art scanning machines in its own Printing House to capture the content of each book selected for inclusion. The files are processed to give a consistently clear, crisp image, and the books finished to the high quality standard for which the Press is recognised around the world. The latest print-on-demand technology ensures that the books will remain available indefinitely, and that orders for single or multiple copies can quickly be supplied.

The Cambridge Library Collection brings back to life books of enduring scholarly value (including out-of-copyright works originally issued by other publishers) across a wide range of disciplines in the humanities and social sciences and in science and technology.

The Works,
Literary, Moral, and Medical,
of Thomas Percival, M.D.

To which are Prefixed,
Memoirs of His Life and Writings,
and a Selection from
His Literary Correspondence

VOLUME 4

THOMAS PERCIVAL

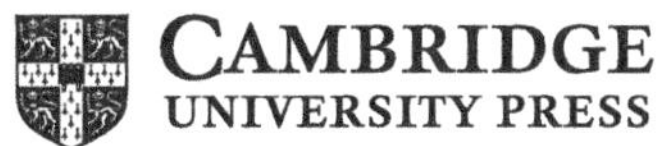

CAMBRIDGE
UNIVERSITY PRESS

University Printing House, Cambridge, CB2 8BS, United Kingdom

Published in the United States of America by Cambridge University Press, New York

Cambridge University Press is part of the University of Cambridge.
It furthers the University's mission by disseminating knowledge in the pursuit of education, learning and research at the highest international levels of excellence.

www.cambridge.org
Information on this title: www.cambridge.org/9781108067362

This edition first published 1807
This digitally printed version 2014

ISBN 978-1-108-06736-2 Paperback

THE

WORKS

OF

THOMAS PERCIVAL, M.D.

IN FOUR VOLUMES.

THE

WORKS,

LITERARY, MORAL,

AND

MEDICAL,

OF

THOMAS PERCIVAL, M.D.

F.R.S. AND A.S.—F.R.S. AND R.M.S. EDIN.

LATE PRES. OF THE LIT. AND PHIL. SOC. AT MANCHESTER; MEMBER OF THE ROYAL SOCIETIES OF PARIS AND OF LYONS, OF THE MEDICAL SOCIETIES OF LONDON, AND OF AIX EN PROVENCE, OF THE AMERIC. ACAD. OF ARTS, &c. AND OF THE AMERIC. PHIL. SOC. AT PHILADELPHIA.

TO WHICH ARE PREFIXED,

MEMOIRS of his LIFE and WRITINGS,

AND A SELECTION FROM HIS

LITERARY CORRESPONDENCE.

A NEW EDITION.

VOL. IV.

PRINTED BY RICHARD CRUTTWELL, ST. JAMES'S-STREET, BATH; FOR J. JOHNSON, ST. PAUL'S CHURCH-YARD, LONDON.

1807.

TO THE REVEREND

THOMAS B. PERCIVAL, LL. B.

OF ST. JOHN'S COLLEGE,

CAMBRIDGE;

WHOSE

MORAL AND INTELLECTUAL ENDOWMENTS

HAVE SUPERADDED

ESTEEM, RESPECT, AND FRIENDSHIP

TO PATERNAL LOVE;

THIS VOLUME

IS

MOST AFFECTIONATELY INSCRIBED

BY

THE AUTHOR.

ESSAYS,

MEDICAL, PHILOSOPHICAL,

AND

EXPERIMENTAL.

ADVERTISEMENT.

THE completion of this volume has been retarded, nearly twelve months, by various causes. It was the author's intention, to have offered the result of his farther experience concerning the HYDROCEPHALUS INTERNUS, *and of the use of* MERCURY *in* AFFECTIONS *of the* HEAD: *And also to have added, to his Remarks on the Improvement of the Manchester Infirmary, some general Observations on the* POLITY OF HOSPITALS. *But he is, at present, too fully occupied with professional and other engagements, to allow due leisure for these undertakings.*

The first, second, and third Parts, into which this work is divided, correspond to the three volumes of former editions. The fourth Part consists of Essays not before comprised in them.

MANCHESTER, OCTOBER 15, 1789.

Lately publiſhed,

BY THE AUTHOR,

New Editions of the following Works, viz.

I. A FATHER's INSTRUCTIONS, conſiſting of MORAL TALES, FABLES, and REFLECTIONS: The ſeventh Edition, reviſed and conſiderably enlarged. Crown 8vo.

II. MORAL and LITERARY DISSERTATIONS, being the SEQUEL TO A FATHER'S INSTRUCTIONS: Second Edition, conſiderably enlarged. Crown 8vo.

THE

CONTENTS.

PART III.

N. B. The additional Essays are marked with an *Asterisk* (*); and those which have been enlarged with a *Dagger* (†).

Miscellaneous

PART IV.

* Narrative

ESSAYS

E S S A Y S

MEDICAL, PHILOSOPHICAL,

AND

EXPERIMENTAL.

PART III.

THE

PREFACE.

IN the Preface to a former volume, publiſhed about three years ago, I availed myſelf of the authority of the great Lord Bacon; whoſe plan I have ſteadily purſued in the collection and arrangement of FACTS, OBSERVATIONS, and EXPERIMENTS. Long and ſyſtematic compoſitions are neither compatible with the extenſive engagements of my profeſſion; nor with the attention which is due from me to a numerous family. But in this deſultory way, I can employ a vacant hour; beguile the diſtance of a tedious journey; or divert the anxieties of a feeling heart, with improvement to myſelf, and, I am willing to hope, with advantage to others.

MANCHESTER, FEB. 6, 1776.

ESSAY

ERRATA.

VOL. I.

Page 37, line 9, for *rifiduum* read *refiduum*. P. 71, note, l. 1, f. *conjuction* r. *conjunction*. P. 83, l. 16. f. *dibilitating* r. *debilitating*. P. 141. note (k), f. *Kaw* r. *Kauw*.

P. 182, l. 1, r. *Eft Elephas morbus, qui propter flumina Nili Gignitur Ægypto in medio.*

P. 191, note (z), f. *Hoffmani* r. *Hoffmanni*. P. 214, note, l. 9, f. *bulkent-felib.* r. *bullient. felib.* P. 237, note (d), f. SCHULTS r. SCHULTZ. P. 294, note, l. 3, f. *it* r. *the preceding obfervations*. P. 377, l. 26, f. *inpervious* r. *impervious*.

VOL. II.

Page 41, note, line 1, f. *Gloucefter* r. *Glocefter*. P. 289, note (a) f. *Heath* r. *Heat*. P. 308, l. 7, f. *But the aftringency, &c.* r. *And the aftringency of it, according to my trials, accompanies its colouring matter*. P. 326, l. 8, f. *trachæa* r. *tracheæ*. P. 380, note (i), l. 4, f. *Vanfwieten* r. *Van Swieten*.

ESSAY I.

OBSERVATIONS ON THE STATE OF POPULATION IN MANCHESTER, AND OTHER ADJACENT PLACES *(a)*.

FROM an account taken in 1717, the number of inhabitants in Manchester, for I am uncertain whether Salford *(b)* was included, appears to have been 8000.

By a survey made in 1757 of Manchester and Salford, the number of inhabitants was

(a) Inserted in the Philosophical Transactions, vols. LXIV. LXV. LXVI.

(b) Manchester and Salford, though distinguished by different names, like London, Westminster, and the Borough of Southwark, may be considered as one and the same town, being divided only by a small river, over which two bridges are erected.

found to be 19839. And from 1754 to 1761 inclufive, the number of deaths amounted to 5769. The annual deaths therefore, at the period of the furvey, muft have been 721, exclufive of diffenters. It is probable, as will appear afterwards, that thefe would have increafed the number to 771. At this time therefore 1 in 25 .7 of the inhabitants of Manchefter died every year.

A NEW furvey of Manchefter has been executed this fummer (1773) with great care and accuracy, of which the following is a particular account.

MANCHESTER.		SALFORD.
3402	Houfes	866.
5317	Families	1099.
10548	Males	2248.
11933	Females	2517.
7724	Married	1775.
432	Widowers	89.
1064	Widows	149.
7782	Under 15	1793.
3252	Above 50	640.
342	Male Lodgers	18.
150	Female ditto	13.
44	Empty Houfes	26.

FROM hence it appears that the number of tenanted houfes in Manchefter and Salford amounts

amounts to 4268; the families to 6416; and the inhabitants to 27,246. The proportion of persons to a house therefore is more than 6⅓; and of individuals to a family about 4¼. The females exceed the males by 1654; the widows are more than double the number of widowers; and about a seventh part of the inhabitants have attained the age of fifty.

The following Table is formed from the Register of Burials and Baptisms at the Collegiate or Parish Church in Manchester, and gives the annual number of each on an average.

			Burials.	Baptisms.
From	1580	to 1587 inclusive,	184	
	1680	1687	286	
	1720	1727	359	
	1754	1760	736	769
	1761	1765	731	843
	1766	1770	870	970

But it should be remarked, that this account does not include the deaths or births amongst the dissenters. These, by a late improvement in our Bills of Mortality, are now received into the Parish Register; and last year (1772) the former amounted to 50, the latter to 181. Admitting these to be the average of unregistered baptisms and burials in Manchester, the annual medium of deaths from 1768 to 1772 inclusive, will

will be 958. And the annual births during the ſame period, with the like allowance, will be 1098. Hence the preſent proportion of annual deaths to the inhabitants is nearly as 1 to 28 4; and of births to the inhabitants almoſt as 1 to 25. The births alſo, it appears, exceed the burials 140 every year at a medium.

THE rapid growth of Mancheſter is ſufficiently evident from the preceding facts. Yet Leverpool, during the ſame ſpace of time, has increaſed in a much greater proportion. This appears from the following Table, which I have extracted from a very curious and entertaining work, lately publiſhed by my ingenious friend the Rev. Dr. Enfield, Lecturer on the Belles Lettres in the Academy at Warrington.

(c) Year.	Number of Inhabitants.	Annual Addition.
1700	5714	
1710	8168	245
1720	10446	227
1730	12074	162
1740	18086	601
1750	22099	401
1760	25787	368
1770	34004	822

(c) Hiſtory of Leverpool, page 28, ſecond edition, corrected.

ACCORDING

According to this Table, Leverpool has at present upwards of six times the number of inhabitants which it contained at the beginning of the century.

But the progress of trade and opulence in Manchester has been more than adequate to its advancement in population. For a considerable part of the manufactory of this flourishing town, is carried on in the adjacent country, which is thereby crowded with houses and inhabitants. So populous are the environs of Manchester, that every house in the township has been found, by a late survey, to contain, at an average, six persons. The township is indeed but of small extent; and the greatest part of it will probably, in a short time, be included in Manchester. It contains 311 houses; 361 families; 947 males; 958 females; 656 married persons; 21 widowers; 42 widows; 763 under 15 years of age; and 222 above 50.

It is pleasing to observe, that, notwithstanding the enlargement of Manchester, there has been a sensible improvement in the healthiness and longevity of its inhabitants; for the proportion of deaths is now considerably less than in 1757. But this is chiefly to be ascribed, as Dr. Price has justly observed *(d)*, to the large accession of

(d) See a most valuable Treatise on Reversionary Payments, p. 188, third edition.

new ſettlers from the country. For as theſe uſually come in the prime of life, they muſt raiſe the proportion of *inhabitants* to the *deaths*, and alſo of *births* and *weddings* to the *burials*, higher than they would otherwiſe be. However, excluſive of this conſideration, there is good reaſon to believe that Mancheſter is more healthy now than formerly. The new ſtreets are wide and ſpacious, the poor have larger and more commodious dwellings, and the increaſe of trade affords them better clothing and diet than they before enjoyed. I may add too, that the late improvements in medicine have been highly favourable to the preſervation of life. The cool regimen in fevers, and in the ſmall-pox; the free admiſſion of air; attention to cleanlineſs; and the general uſe of antiſeptic remedies and diet, have certainly mitigated the violence, and leſſened the mortality of ſome of the moſt dangerous and malignant diſtempers to which mankind are incident. The ulcerous ſore throat, which prevailed here in the year 1770, is the only epidemic which has appeared in Mancheſter, with any fatal degree of violence, for many years. Miliary fevers, which were formerly frequent in this town and neighbourhood, now rarely occur; and if I may judge from my own experience, the natural ſmall-pox (for inoculation is not much practiſed here) carries off a ſmaller proportion of thoſe

who

who are attacked by it, than is commonly ſuppoſed. Puerperal diſeaſes alſo decreaſe every year amongſt us, by the judicious method of treating women in child-bed: and as nature is now more conſulted in the management of infants, it is reaſonable to ſuppoſe that this muſt be favourable to their health and preſervation.

But it muſt be acknowledged that large towns are injurious to population; and the advantages I have enumerated, which in hamlets or country villages would have operated with full force to the benefit of mankind, have only ſerved to check the deſtructive tendency of the accumulation of inhabitants in Mancheſter. In the Pais de Vaud, a diſtrict of the province of Bern in Switzerland, and in a country pariſh in Brandenburgh, 1 in 45 of the inhabitants die annually; and at Stoke Damarell in Devonſhire, 1 in 54 *(e)*: whereas in this town the yearly mortality appears to be 1 in 28; in Leverpool 1 in 27; and in London 1 in 21. Half the children who are born in Mancheſter die under five years old; and the proportion which the births bear to the number of inhabitants who attain the age of 80, is as 30 to 1. Diſeaſes are moſt frequent and fatal here in the months of January, February, and March; and

(e) See the Treatiſe before referred to, on Reverſionary Payments, by my learned friend Dr. Price.

leaſt ſo in July, Auguſt, and September. The mortality of theſe two ſeaſons is as 11 to 8; and of the firſt ſix months of the year compared with the laſt ſix months, as 7 to 6.

In April, 1773, ſeveral gentlemen, from motives of curioſity, undertook an enumeration of the people of Bolton, a manufacturing town about twelve miles diſtant from Mancheſter. The houſes were found to be 946; the males 2159; the females 2392; and perſons aged ſeventy years and upwards, 74. To theſe numbers 17 muſt be added, which by a miſtake were not claſſed under either denomination. The inhabitants of Bolton therefore amount to 4568; the number of individuals to a houſe is 4 .8; and about a ſixtieth part of the people have attained the age of ſeventy.

Little Bolton, a ſuburb of Bolton, including the manor, and extending into the country as far as the inhabitants are ſubject to *ſuit* and *ſervice*, contains 232 houſes; 771 individuals; 361 males; 410 females; and 15 perſons aged ſeventy years and upwards. From this account it appears that the inhabitants are 3 .3 to a houſe; and that 1 in 51 has reached the age of ſeventy. The difference in theſe proportions between a ſmall *town*, and a *country manor* contiguous to it, is worthy of obſervation.

Mr.

Mr. Fletcher has favoured me with an enumeration of the people of Bury, which he has juſt executed with great care. The town contains 463 houſes; 464 families; and 2090 inhabitants. Each houſe and family therefore conſiſts of 4½ individuals. Bury is ſituated nine miles from Mancheſter, and is enriched by a branch of the woollen manufactory.

At Altringham, a market town in Cheſhire, which has no manufactory, the number of houſes, according to an exact ſurvey made in July, 1772, was 248; of inhabitants 1029, or $4\frac{1}{7}$ to a houſe. An enumeration of the people of this town was made about twenty years ago, at which time they amounted very nearly to 1000.

The following is a comparative view of the ſtate of population, the duration of life, and the mortality of the ſeveral ſeaſons of the year, &c. in Eastham, and Royton, two country places widely different from each other in climate, ſituation, and in the occupation of their inhabitants.

The pariſh of Eaſtham lies in Wirral, one of the hundreds into which Cheſhire is divided, and is extended along the banks of the river Merſey, a few miles diſtant from the Iriſh ſea. The people are moſt of them farmers; though ſome are fiſhermen, and others are employed in the ferry to Leverpool.

Royton

Royton is a chapelry, ſituated ten miles eaſtward of Mancheſter, under the great chain of mountains which divides Lancaſhire and Yorkſhire. The inhabitants are employed chiefly in the cotton and linen manufactory; a few of them are farmers; and ſome I believe work in the coal pits, with which this country abounds.

I am indebted to my learned friend the Rev. Mr. Travis, Vicar of Eaſtham, for the ſurvey of his own pariſh, which he undertook at my deſire, and executed himſelf; and alſo for that of Royton, which was made by his uncle, the worthy and reſpectable clergyman of that chapelry.

JANUARY 1ft, 1772, the number of inhabitants in the chapelry of Royton were found to be 1105.

The number of inhabitants in the parifh of Eaftham, 912.

The number of perfons *in a houfe*, in the chapelry of Royton is fomewhat more than - - - $5\frac{1}{7}$.
The number of ditto, - in the parifh of Eaftham, - - - exactly - - - 5.
The number of perfons *in a family*, in the former, on an average, - - about - - - $4\frac{3}{4}$.
The number of ditto, - in the latter, - - - - - more than - - $4\frac{1}{2}$.
The proportion of males to females, in Royton, - - - - - nearly as - 53 to 56.
The proportion of ditto, - in Eaftham, - - - - - nearly as - $54\frac{1}{2}$ to 56.
The widows to the widowers, - in Royton, - - - - - as - - - $3\frac{1}{3}$ to 1.
The widows ditto, - in Eaftham, - - - - - as - - - 3 to $2\frac{1}{2}$.
The number of births in Royton (on an average of 3 years) 42. } Proportion between males and females as 13 to 11.
The number of ditto, - in Eaftham ditto, 34. } Proportion between ditto, - as 18 to 16.
N. B. Thefe proportions for 7 years.

The number of births in Royton to the number of married inhabitants, as (very nearly) 1 child to 5 married couples.
The number of do. in Eaftham to ditto, - - as (fomewhat more than) 1 child to 4 married couples.
The number of births in Royton to the whole number of inhabitants, - - as - - 1 to $26\frac{1}{3}$.
The number of do. in Eaftham to ditto, - - - - - - as - - 1 to $26\frac{4}{5}$.
The number of married perfons in Royton to the number of unmarried perfons above 15, - as - 8 to 5.
The number of ditto, - in Eaftham to the number of - ditto, - ditto, - nearly as 6 to 5.

The number of burials in Royton (on an average of 3 years) 21. } Proportion between males and females as 13 to 10.
The number of ditto in Eaſtham - ditto - 26. } Proportion between - ditto - as 14 to 12.
The number of burials in Royton to the number of all the inhabitants, - as - 1 to 52.
The number of ditto in Eaſtham to - ditto, - - - - as - 1 to 35.
The number of children dying under 3 yrs. old to the number of children born in Royton (on an average of 3 yrs.) as 1 to 7.
The number of children - ditto - to - ditto - in Eaſtham - - as 1 to 17.
Perſons alive in Royton under 3 years old Jan. 1, 1772, 129; dead under 3 years old, average of 3 years, 6, or 1 of $21\frac{1}{2}$.
Ditto in Eaſtham - - - - 100; - - - - - dead 2, or 1 of 50.
Perſons alive in Royton under 15 years old Jan. 1, 1772, 450; dead under 15 years old, average of 3 years, 11, or 1 of 41.
Ditto in Eaſtham - - - - 329; - - - dead 4, or 1 of 82.
Perſons alive in Royton between 15 and 30 years old Jan. 1, 1772, 333; dead before 1773 of theſe 5, or 1 of $66\frac{1}{2}$.
Ditto in Eaſtham - - - - 199; - - dead 5, or 1 of 40.
Perſons alive in Royton from 30 to 40 years old ditto, 96; dead before 1773 of theſe on an average, 2, or 1 of 48.
Ditto in Eaſtham - - - - 124; - - - dead 4, or 1 of 31.
Perſons alive in Royton from 40 to 50 years old ditto, 98; dead before 1773 of theſe on an average, 2, or 1 of 49.
Ditto in Eaſtham - - - 83; dead before 1773 of theſe - 3, or 1 of 28.
Perſons alive in Royton from 50 to 60 years old ditto, 61; dead before 1773 of theſe - $1\frac{1}{3}$, or 1 of 45.
Ditto in Eaſtham - - - 64; dead before 1773 of theſe - 2, or 1 of 32.

Perſons alive in Royton from 60 to 70 years old ditto, 49; dead before 1773 of theſe - - $1\frac{1}{3}$, or 1 of 36.

Ditto in Eaſtham - - - 54; deád before 1773 of theſe - - $1\frac{1}{3}$, or 1 of 40.

Perſons alive in Royton from 70 to 80,	Jan. 1, 1772,	10	above 70 years, 18	dead before 1773, on an average of 3 years,	1 of 18.
80 to 90,	ditto,	8			
Perſons alive in Eaſtham from 70 to 80,	ditto,	34	above 70 years, 39	dead before 1773, on an average of 3 years,	1 of 21.
80 to 90,	ditto,	5			(*f*)

The mortality of the ſeaſons at Royton and Eaſtham, for the laſt ſeven years, has been as follows:

			ROYTON.	EASTHAM.
January,	February,	March,	39	56
April,	May,	June,	31	34
July,	Auguſt,	September,	31	45
October,	November,	December,	18	53
			119	188

(*f*) The averages here adopted may, in ſome inſtances, ſeem to be too ſmall; but Mr. Travis aſſures me, that through a ſeries of fifteen ſucceſſive years, the marriages, births, and deaths at Eaſtham, do not vary, in any degree worth remarking, from the foregoing table.

Of all the months in the year ſingly taken, October is the moſt, and April the leaſt fatal to the inhabitants of Eaſtham. Whereas the three laſt months of the year appear to be the moſt healthful at Royton; although a very large quantity of rain uſually falls there during this ſeaſon. For the wind at this time being generally weſterly, the clouds are intercepted by the high mountains, and diſcharge themſelves in frequent and heavy ſhowers. At Townley, which is ſituated under the ſame chain of hills, and is not very far diſtant from Royton, 42 inches of rain fall at a medium, every year. The quantity of rain at Mancheſter, which is farther removed from the mountains, is about 33 inches *communibus annis* (g). It has been obſerved by a very uſeful writer, that the *moiſt ſeaſons* in Great Britain and Ireland are more remarkably free from epidemic diſeaſes, than the dry ones; and that ſtorms, the uſual concomitants of rain, are attended with more health and leſs ſickneſs than calm weather, probably becauſe they diſſipate the vapours, which by ſtagnation might prove an occaſion of various diſtem-

(g) The rain-gauge at Townley appears to have been placed on the top of the houſe; whereas, at Mancheſter, this inſtrument was very near the ground. It is evident, therefore, that the diſparity muſt be eſtimated at much more than nine inches.

pers

" Perhaps ſuch a regulation is ſcarcely practica-
" ble with us."

But an enumeration of the people of England, ſimilar to that lately executed at Mancheſter, would not be ſo difficult an undertaking, as may at the firſt view be imagined. And if accurate, and comprehenſive Bills of Mortality were univerſally eſtabliſhed, they would admirably coincide with the views of ſuch inquiries, and give preciſion and certainty to the concluſions deduced from them *(b)*.

From the populouſneſs of this neighbourhood, it may perhaps be ſuppoſed, that a great number of burials are brought from the country to the collegiate and other churches in Mancheſter, and that this circumſtance is likely to create uncertainty and error in the calculations made from the parochial regiſter of deaths. But it appears, from the beſt information I can collect, that the number of ſuch burials is not conſiderable; and that they are pretty exactly balanced by thoſe which are carried out of Mancheſter to the neighbouring epiſcopal or diſſenting chapels. This fact admits of an eaſy and ſatisfactory

(b) See Propoſals for eſtabliſhing accurate Bills of Mortality in Mancheſter, vol. I. p. 428. Theſe Propoſals have been adopted, and, with a few variations, carried into execution by Dr. Haygarth at Cheſter, Dr. Dobſon at Leverpool, and by Mr. John Aikin at Warrington.

 explanation,

explanation, were it neceſſary to trouble the reader with it.

It is remarked, in the former paper, that wet ſeaſons are generally more free from epidemic diſeaſes than dry ones, and the Bills of Mortality at Mancheſter *ſeem* to confirm the obſervation: It appears at leaſt from the following table, that the year 1766, remarkable in this climate for the ſmall quantity of rain which fell during the courſe of it, was more fatal than any of the reſt. And the proportion of deaths will be deemed greater, when it is recollected, that the town contained at that time fewer inhabitants probably, by two thouſand, than it does at preſent. For the rapid increaſe of Mancheſter commenced about the year 1765, after the concluſion of the laſt war.

Year.	Quantity of Rain at Mancheſter. Inches.	Deaths at Mancheſter.
1765	31. 378	723
1766	25. 762	1019
1767	29. 186	690
1768	40. 526	867
1769	32. 514	788
1770	39. 363	988
1771 from Jan. 1. to June 1.	6. 8 (c)	

This

(c) This account of the quantity of rain, was communicated to me by George Lloyd, Eſq. F.R.S. The obſervations

This table, it muft be acknowledged, does not comprehend a fufficient length of time to

tions were made at his feat, about a mile diftant from the centre of Manchefter, and were continued only till June 1771.

The following is an abridged view of a meteorological regifter, which I kept, with great exactnefs, during the years 1774 and 1775.

Months.	Thermometer. Two o'Clock P. M. Higheft.	Loweft.	Days. Rainy.	Dry.
	1774.			
Jan. Feb. March,	56.	28.	25.	65.
April, May, June,	72.	45.	55.	36.
July, Aug. Sept.	75.	53.	66.	26.
Oct. Nov. Dec.	60.	30.	43.	49.
Mean heat	52,25.		189.	176.
	1775.			
Jan. Feb. March,	54.	30.	61.	29.
April, May, June,	78.	51.	42.	49.
July, Aug. Sept.	74.	48.	62.	30.
Oct. Nov. Dec.	64.	32.	50.	28.
Mean heat	55,7		215.	136.

N. B. In 1775, fourteen days are omitted, no account being taken.

The thermometer was made by Dollond, and graduated according to the fcale of Fahrenheit. It was placed in the open air, and in a northern expofure. The column of rainy days expreffes the *leaft*, as well as the *greateft* quantity of rain; the column of days includes only thofe days, in which not a fingle fhower was noticed. The day comprehends twenty-four hours.

 admit

admit of any very accurate or incontrovertible conclusions. And the influence of other causes of disease, which have little or no relation to the state of the atmosphere, together with the irregularity which necessarily occurs in the annual increase of a large manufacturing town, may be regarded as farther sources of fallacy and uncertainty. It is therefore with diffidence I observe, that though wet seasons are less mortal than long continued droughts, yet the rainy years 1768 and 1770 proved extremely sickly and fatal. And those years are probably most unfavourable to health, in which heavy rains fall about the beginning of summer, and are succeeded by great and uninterrupted heats. For the earth being thus drenched with moisture, and the low lands overflowed with water, the exhalations become constant, copious, and often putrid.

JOAN LEO in his history of Africa relates, that if heavy rains fall in that country during the months of July and August, the plague usually breaks out the September following *(d)*. But in European climates, it is well remarked by Sir John Pringle, that frequent showers in summer cool the air, check the excess of vapour, dilute and refresh the corrupted waters,

(d) Hist. Africæ, lib. I. cap. 10.

and precipitate the noxious effluvia which float in the atmofphere *(e)*. And it appears, from a variety of obfervations which I have collected, that October, November, and December are generally very healthy, although the moft rainy months in the year. I fhall fubjoin a table which will fet this point in the cleareft light; and at the fame time fhew the comparative mortality of the different feafons at Middleton, Bowden, Chowbent, Difhley, Middlewich, Richmond, and Manchefter. *(f)*

(e) See Sir John Pringle on the Difeafes of the Army, p. 5, edit. fourth.

(f) Extract of a letter from Dr. Farr, dated April 13, 1782.

" Before I left the Briftol Infirmary, I took an ac-" count of all the difeafes which occurred in it for a number " of years; and as all acute cafes are admitted, it is, in " general, an epitome of the ftate of difeafes in the town. " I have fent you an account for three years, during which " time I kept a regifter of the rain."

	1775	1776	1777
Synochus - - -	166	95	137
Typhus - - -	35	21	33
Intermittents - -	16	14	4
Pleurifies and Peripneumonies	20	43	25
Inflammations - -	8	15	18
Acute Rheumatifm - -	52	66	64
	297	254	281
Rain. Inches, - -	38,597,	28,554,	23,369

A TABLE shewing the COMPARATIVE MORTALITY of the different SEASONS of the YEAR.

	Middleton from 1663 to 1673 Ten years.	Middleton from 1763 to 1773. Ten years.	Bowden from 1663 to 1673. Ten years.	Bowden from 1763 to 1773. Ten years.	Manchester from 1766 to 1774.* Eight years.
January, February, March,	117.	265.	179.	259.	1538.
April, May, June,	99.	291.	139.	300.	1366.
July, August, September,	79.	215.	114.	209.	957.
October, November, December.	72.	222.	127.	207.	1339.

* This account is taken from the register of the collegiate or parish church only.

Chowbent

	Chowbent from 1767 to 1773. Six years.	Difhley from 1763 to 1773. Ten years.	Middlewich from 1768 to 1773. Five years.	Richmond from 1764 to 1774. Ten years.	Rochdale from 1760 to 1773. Thirteen years.
January, February, March,	71.	64.	67.	170.	1533.
April, May, June,	37.	78.	55.	156.	1336.
July, Auguft, September,	28.	51.	59.	172.	1077.
October, November, December.	33.	43.	69.	144.	1239.

Total.

Total.	Jan.	Feb.	March,	4263.
	April,	May,	June,	3857.
	July,	Aug.	Sep.	2961.
	Oct.	Nov.	Dec.	3495.

THERE is a conſiderable diverſity in the ſituation of theſe places. Middleton lies ſix miles north eaſt of Mancheſter, not far from the great chain of mountains which divides Lancaſhire and Yorkſhire; and about thirty-ſix miles from the ſea.

BOWDEN is ten miles to the ſouth weſt of Mancheſter, and thirty-five miles from the ſea. It is an elevated ſituation, in a level country; and at a great diſtance from any hills.

CHOWBENT is ten miles weſtward of Mancheſter, and twenty five miles diſtant from the ſea. It is in a low and flat ſituation, and near a very extenſive moraſs.

DISHLEY is in that part of Cheſhire, which borders on the peak of Derbyſhire. It is a mountainous ſituation, thirteen miles ſouth eaſt of Mancheſter, and fifty miles from the ſea.

MIDDLEWICH is twenty eight miles ſouthward of Mancheſter, and about forty miles from the ſea. It is ſurrounded by a well cultivated and level country.

RICHMOND is a conſiderable market town in the north riding of Yorkſhire, about forty miles diſtant

diſtant from the German ocean. It ſtands on an eminence, which terminates a long continued range of mountains. The country below is an extenſive, rich, and well cultivated plain.

THE obſervations of Dr. Franklin on the ſubject of moiſture will, I doubt not, be very acceptable to the medical reader, although he may not entirely acquieſce in the opinion of this excellent philoſopher. I ſhall therefore give a farther quotation from the letter before referred to. "The gentry of England are remarkably "afraid of moiſture, and of air. But ſeamen, "who live in perpetually moiſt air, are always "healthy if they have good proviſions. The "inhabitants of Bermudas, St. Heſen, and other "iſlands far from continents, ſurrounded with "rocks, againſt which the waves continually "daſhing fill the air with ſpray and vapour, and "where no wind can ariſe that does not paſs "over much ſea, and of courſe bring much "moiſture, are remarkably healthy. And I "have long thought, mere moiſt air has no ill "effect on the conſtitution; though air impregnated with vapours from putrid marſhes is "found pernicious, not from its moiſture, but "putridity. It ſeems ſtrange that a man, whoſe "body is compoſed in great part of moiſt fluids, "whoſe blood and juices are ſo watery, who can "ſwallow quantities of water and ſmall beer

" daily, without inconvenience, ſhould fancy that " a little more or leſs moiſture in the air ſhould " be of ſuch importance. But we abound in " abſurdity and inconſiſtency."

In the former paper, I gave a ſtriking example of the great advantages of diligence and ſobriety, in *the length of days* which the people of Monton enjoy. Such an inſtance, though a ſingle one, affords the moſt animating leſſon of morality; and I can enforce it by farther proofs.

The Rev. Mr. Harrop has favoured me with an account of the people who attend divine ſervice in the chapel at Hale, near Altringham, which he has lately taken, with a retroſpect of the births and deaths amongſt them during the laſt ſeven years. The ſociety is compoſed of 140 males, 136 females, 92 married perſons, 8 widowers, 12 widows, 105 under fifteen years of age, and 41 above fifty. The deaths during ſeven years have been 28, and the births 68. It appears from this enumeration, that only one in 69 of the people, who are moſt of them farmers, dies annually. Hale is a low ſituation, and the ſoil is clayey.

The congregration belonging to the chapel at Horwich conſiſts of 305 individuals, viz. 149 males, and 156 females, 94 married perſons, and 9 widowers, 8 widows, 127 under fifteen years of age, and 50 above fifty. The births for the laſt

ſeven

ſeven years have amounted to 101, and the deaths to 32. Hence the yearly proportion of deaths to the inhabitants is as 1 to 66. Horwich is between Bolton and Chorley, the country is mountainous, and the people are compoſed almoſt equally of farmers and manufacturers. I am obliged to the Rev. Mr. Evans for this account.

THE Rev. Mr. Smalley of Darwen, three miles from Blackburn in Lancaſhire, has tranſmitted to me the following ſurvey of his congregation. It conſiſts of 1850 individuals; 900 males; 950 females; 640 married perſons; 30 widowers; 48 widows; 737 perſons under the age of fifteen, and 218 above fifty. During the laſt ſeven years the deaths have amounted to 233; and the births to 508. The annual proportion of deaths therefore is 1 in 56; and the births are to the number of inhabitants nearly as 1 to 25 .5. Darwen is a country diſtrict, bleak and elevated in its ſituation, ſurrounded by moors, and ill cultivated. The inhabitants are chiefly employed in the cotton manufactory.

A CLERGYMAN in the peak of Derbyſhire has, at my deſire, undertaken an enumeration of the people of Edale, a fertile valley in that part of the county, inhabited by a ſober and induſtrious race of farmers. But I have not yet received a particular account of the ſurvey; and have only been

been informed, that 1 in 59 of the inhabitants dies annually, on an average of ten years.

The principles and manners of the Quakers, though often made the ſubjects of illiberal cenſure and ridicule, may probably afford them advantages, with reſpect to the duration of life, over other bodies of men. The diligence, cleanlineſs, temperance and compoſure of mind, by which the members of this ſociety are in general diſtinguiſhed, may reaſonably be ſuppoſed to contribute to health and longevity: And as there are no perſons among them in abject poverty, and few immoderately rich, this more equal diſtribution of property muſt leſſen the ſources of diſeaſe, and furniſh every individual under it with the neceſſary means of relief. Theſe conſiderations excited my curioſity to know the proportion of deaths amongſt the Quakers in Mancheſter; and I have been gratified by Mr. Routh, in the moſt obliging manner, with the following information. The ſociety conſiſts of 81 males; and 84 females; 54 married perſons; 9 widowers; 7 widows; and 48 perſons under fifteen years of age. The births during the laſt ſeven years have amounted to 34; and the burials to 47. About 1 therefore in 24.6 of the Quakers in Mancheſter dies annually; whereas the proportion of deaths amongſt the inhabitants of the town at large is as 1 to 28. If no allowance be made for the temporary and accidental irregularities which may occur in a ſingle and ſmall body of men, when the average of a few years has only been taken, a concluſion directly contrary to what I have preſuppoſed, will be drawn from this fact. And perhaps it will be urged, that the want of vivacity in the people of this ſect, and the ſedentary lives of their females, are cauſes which ſhorten the period of their exiſtence, and counterbalance the advantages from cleanlineſs and ſobriety, which they enjoy. But the reader will entertain a different opinion concerning this point, when he is informed, that the Quakers here have had few or no acceſſions to their number, by ſupplies from other places, during the laſt ſeven years. This muſt conſiderably increaſe their proportional mortality, for reaſons which have been before aſſigned; and is the true cauſe, why the deaths amongſt them ſo much exceed the births. Were it not for new ſettlers in the prime of life, who annually pour into Mancheſter, it is probable that more than 1 in 25 of its inhabitants would die annually. So baleful is the influence of large towns on the duration of life; and ſo juſtly are they ſtiled, by a writer of the moſt diſtinguiſhed abilities, the *graves* of mankind (*g*)!

(*g*) Dr. Price.

THE

The Rev. Mr. Barnes, whom I cannot mention without expreſſions of eſteem and friendſhip, made a ſurvey in September, 1773, of the people belonging to the new chapel at Cockey Moor, near Bolton, the particulars of which are as follow:

Houſes	150.
Families	154.
Males	320.
Females	391.
Married perſons	248.
Widowers	10.
Widows	27.
Under fifteen	252.
Above fifty	99.
Births in five years	125.
Deaths in ſeven years	114.
Total number of people	711.

The married perſons in this ſociety are therefore to the ſingle as 1 to 1 .867; the widows are nearly treble the number of widowers; a ſeventh part of the people have attained the age of fifty, and thoſe under fifteen exceed one third of the whole congregation. The average number of births is 25 every year, and of deaths $16\frac{2}{7}$; ſo that the former are to the latter, in the proportion of ſomewhat more than 5 to 3; and 1 perſon

ſon in about 44 dies annually. It ſhould be remarked, that the number of deaths in this period was conſiderably increaſed by the uncommon fatality of the ſmall-pox in the year 1770. Cockey Moor is ſurrounded by a cold, wet, and barren country; the inhabitants are farmers and manufacturers.

The congregation belonging to the chapel at Chowbent conſiſts of 1160 perſons, viz. 554 males; 606 females; 173 males, and 150 females under 10 years of age; 83 males, and 91 females above fifty; 6 males, and 4 females above eighty; 199 married couples; 26 widowers; and 43 widows. The baptiſms during ſix years (wanting ſix weeks) have amounted to 293; and the deaths to 169. About 1 therefore in 41 .2 of this ſociety dies annually. This ſurvey was made in November, 1773, by the Rev. Mr. Mercer. The people of Chowbent are employed chiefly in the manufactories of cotton, linen, and iron.

At Ackworth, near Ferry-bridge in the county of York, the chriſtenings and burials for ten years, viz. from March 25th 1757, to March 25th 1767, have been as follow:

Christenings.		Burials.	
Males	104.	Males.	79.
Females	108.	Females	77.
Total	212.	Total	156.

Of this number have died,

	Males.	Females.	Total.
Under 2 years old	18	13	31
Between 2 and 5	9	7	16
5 and 10	4	1	5
10 and 20	2	2	4
20 and 30	7	5	12
30 and 40	3	8	11
40 and 50	2	4	6
50 and 60	11	3	14
60 and 70	13	13	26
70 and 80	7	14	21
80 and 90	3	6	9
90 and 100	0	1	1
Of all ages in ten years	79	77	156

Diseases.	Males.	Females.	Total.
Child-bed	0	2	2
Chincough	0	2	2
Confumption	23	15	38
Diabetes	1	0	1
Fever	12	11	23
Infants	7	6	13
Meafles	0	2	2
Old Age	11	19	30
Small Pox	7	6	13
Dyfentery	1	1	2
Dropfy	0	3	3
Apoplexy	2	1	3

In

In this pariſh there are,

184 Houſes, eleven of which are uninhabited.

728 Perſons, of the following ages, viz.

	Males.	Females.	Total.
Under 2 Years old	31	25	56
Between 2 and 5	32	36	68
5 and 10	34	38	72
10 and 20	50	51	101
20 and 30	44	63	107
30 and 40	61	62	123
40 and 50	31	38	69
50 and 60	28	32	60
60 and 70	20	28	48
70 and 80	7	10	17
80 and 90	2	4	6
90 and 100	0	1	1
Of all ages—Total	340	388	

This account of Ackworth was lately tranſmitted to my friend Mr. White, by the Rev. Dr. Lee, Rector of the pariſh. It appears that 1 in 46 .6 of the inhabitants dies yearly; and that the proportion of perſons to each tenanted houſe is 4 $\frac{1}{5}$. Amongſt the males under 2 years of age, the number of deaths exceeds, by a third, thoſe amongſt the females; and 43 women and only 29 men have attained the age

 of

of ſixty and upwards. Theſe facts (and I could adduce many ſimilar ones) confirm a curious remark lately advanced by Dr. Price, that the life of males is more frail than that of females.

I SHALL conclude this Paper with a Table deduced from the preceding obſervations.

FEB. 1ſt, 1774.

A TABLE

A TABLE shewing the PROPORTION of INHABITANTS *dying annually* in feveral different Places.

MANCHESTER.	LEVERPOOL.	CHOWBENT.	EASTHAM.	COCKEY.	ROYTON.
1. in 28.	1. in 27 ·7.	1. in 41.	1. in 35.	1. in 44.	1. in 52.
DARWEN.	EDALE.	ACKWORTH.	HORWICH.	HALE.	MONTON.
1. in 56.	1. in 59.	1. in 47.	1. in 66.	1. in 69.	1. in 68.

OBSERVATIONS

ON THE

STATE *of* POPULATION *in* MANCHESTER, *and other* ADJACENT PLACES, *concluded.*

A VERY accurate ſurvey was completed laſt year of the towns of Mancheſter and Salford, with their reſpective townſhips. This ſpring an enumeration, equally exact and comprehenſive, has been made of the whole pariſh of Mancheſter; which contains thirty-one townſhips (excluſive of the two above-mentioned) in the compaſs of leſs than ſixty ſquare miles. The reader is here preſented with the particulars of this enumeration.

Tenanted houſes	2371.
Families	2525.
Inhabitants	13,786.
Males	6942.
Females	6844.
Married	4319.
Widowers	232.
Widows	315.
Under fifteen	5545.
Above fifty	1762.
Above ſixty	470.

Above

Above ſeventy	261.
Above eighty	87.
Male lodgers	68.
Female lodgers	51.
Empty houſes	41.

THE number of perſons to a houſe, in the pariſh of Mancheſter, is therefore nearly $5\frac{4}{5}$; of individuals to a family about $5\frac{1}{2}$; and $\frac{1}{5}$th of the inhabitants have attained the age of fifty. It is unneceſſary to point out the difference in the proportions between the *town* and adjacent *country*, as it will appear ſufficiently obvious, by comparing this account with that of Mancheſter. The whole number of inhabitants in the town, townſhip, and pariſh of Mancheſter, amounts to 42937.

AT the cloſe of 1772, an account was collected from every country chapel, both Epiſcopal and Diſſenting, in the pariſh, of the baptiſms and burials of that year. The former were found to amount to 401; the latter to 246; and there is a preſumption, that this is nearly the annual proportion of deaths in the pariſh of Mancheſter, excluſive of the town and townſhip. For the number of burials in the whole pariſh was, in the ſame year, exactly 1200; and it has been ſhewn, that the deaths in the town of Mancheſter are, one year with another,

 958.

958. This ſum being ſubtracted from 1200, leaves a remainder (242) for the country, very nearly equal to 246. And if 13786, the number of people in the pariſh, be divided by 246, it will appear that only one in 56 of the inhabitants dies annually; whilſt the yearly mortality in Mancheſter is as 1 to 28. Such a ſtriking diſparity in the healthineſs of a large town, and of the country which ſurrounds it, granting it to be leſs than has been ſuppoſed, will ſcarcely be credited by thoſe, who have paid no attention to inquiries of this nature. And it muſt afford matter of aſtoniſhment even to the phyſician and philoſopher, when he reflects, that the inhabitants of both live in the ſame climate, carry on the ſame manufactures, and are chiefly ſupplied with proviſions from the ſame market. But his ſurpriſe will give place to concern and regret, when he obſerves the havoc produced in every large town by luxury, irregularity, and intemperance *(a)*; the numbers that fall annual

(a) THERE are at this time, in Mancheſter, no leſs than 193 licenſed houſes for retailing ſpirituous and other liquors; and 64 in the other townſhips of the pariſh. At Birmingham, the number of public houſes is ſtill greater than at Mancheſter. A very ingenious friend of mine in that place has computed, that the quantity of malt conſumed there in the public houſes, requires for its growth, a compaſs of land which would be ſufficient for the ſupport of 20,000 men.

victims

victims to the contagious diſtempers, which never ceaſe to prevail; and the pernicious influence of confinement, uncleanlineſs, and foul air on the duration of life *(b)*.

> Ye who amid this feveriſh world would wear
> A body free of pain, of cares a mind;
> Fly the rank city, ſhun its turbid air;
> Breathe not the chaos of eternal ſmoke
> And volatile corruption, from the dead,
> The dying, ſickening, and the living world
> Exhaled, to ſully heaven's tranſparent dome
> With dim mortality.
>
> *Armſtrong on Health*, Book I.

GREAT towns are in a peculiar degree fatal to children. Half of all that are born in London die under two, and in Mancheſter under five years of age; whereas at Royton, a country townſhip not far diſtant from Mancheſter, the number of children dying under the age of three years, is to the number of children born only as 1 to 7: and at Eaſtham, a pariſh in Cheſhire inhabited by farmers, the proportion is conſiderably leſs.

IT is a common, but injurious practice, in manufacturing countries, to confine children, before

(b) THE Rev. Dr. Tucker, Dean of Glouceſter, informs me, "That were it not for the daily arrival of recruits from "the country, his pariſh (St. Stephens, in Briſtol) and in- "deed Briſtol in general, would be left in a century without "an inhabitant; unleſs the people ſhould betake themſelves "to better courſes."

they

they have attained a ſufficient degree of ſtrength, to ſedentary employments, in places where they breathe a putrid air, and are debarred the free uſe of their limbs. The effect of this confinement, ſays an able writer, is either to cut them off early in life, or to render their conſtitutions feeble and ſickly. But the love of money ſtifles the feelings of humanity, and even makes men blind to the very intereſt they ſo anxiouſly purſue. The ſame principle of ſound policy, which induces them to ſpare their horſes and cattle, till they arrive at a due ſize and vigour, ſhould determine them to grant a proportionable reſpite to their children *(c)*. And this obſervation may, perhaps, be extended to the untimely culture of the mind. For too early an application to ſtudy impairs the faculties, injures the conſtitution, and hurts the temper by frequent contradiction. Almoſt as ſoon as a boy has acquired the powers of ſpeech, he is ſhut up many hours every day in a noiſome ſchool, ſecluded from the benefit of exerciſe and the refreſhment of the open air, and tied down to the ſevere drudgery of learning what ſerves only, at ſuch a period of life, to overcharge his memory, and to deſtroy his native cheerfulneſs of diſpoſition. Thus the age of gaiety (to uſe the

(c) See Dr. Gregory's Comparative View of the State and Faculties of Man, &c.

words

words of the elegant writer before referred to) is ſpent in the midſt of tears, puniſhments, and ſlavery; and this to anſwer no other end but to make a child a man, ſome years before nature intended he ſhould be one.

The Rev. Mr. Harriſon of Chapel in le Frith has made a ſurvey, at my requeſt, of the inhabitants of Chinley, Brownſide, and Bugſworth; three hamlets contiguous to each other, in the pariſh of Gloſſop, and peak of Derbyſhire. They are four ſtatute miles in length, and three in breadth; and contain 301 males; 310 females; 200 married perſons; 15 widowers; 18 widows; 234 perſons under fifteen years of age; 121 above fifty; and 9 who have attained the age of eighty. This enumeration was finiſhed in September, 1773.

I have been furniſhed by the Rev. Mr. Aſsheton, Rector of Middleton near Mancheſter, with an account of the births, deaths, and marriages in his pariſh, during ten correſponding years of the laſt, and of the preſent century. From 1663 to 1672 incluſive, the deaths were, males 180, females 187; the births, males 200, females 188; the marriages 121.

The births therefore, during ten years, only exceeded the deaths in number 21; and the average number of births to each marriage, was as $3\frac{1}{5}$ to 1.

From

From 1763 to 1772 inclusive, the deaths were, 499 males, 494 females; the christenings, 802 males, 768 females; the marriages 330. The baptisms therefore, during this period, exceeded the deaths 577, that is, near 58 annually. And if no allowance be made for illegitimate births (which, I believe, in this parish are not numerous, and can no where be supposed equal to one fourth of all that are born) each marriage has produced 4¾ children.

It is curious to observe the change both in the proportion of births to the deaths, and also to the marriages, which has taken place at Middleton (and I have received similar accounts of other places) during the course of the last century. The former may be explained by the greater encouragement to matrimony, from the increase of trade: The latter is of more difficult solution; though it is probable that the warmer cloathing, and better fare, which the poor now enjoy, may have contributed to it. Luxury, when carried to such a degree as to enervate the constitution, is unfavourable to population; but plenty of nutritive diet may well be regarded as a source of fruitfulness. The lower class of people, in this country, formerly lived upon the coarsest food. Wheat, an hundred years ago, was almost unknown to them; and so lately has it been cultivated in Lancashire, that it has scarcely yet acquired the name of corn,

corn, which in general is applied only to barley, oats, and rye. Potatoes alſo are much improved by the preſent judicious method of growing and propagating them; and they now conſtitute a moſt wholeſome and nouriſhing part of our diet.

A PHYSICIAN, of the firſt rank in his profeſſion, has ſuggeſted to me, that tea may be conſidered as a powerful aphrodiſiac; and he imputes the amazing population of China, amongſt other cauſes, to the general uſe of it. But the Dutch, who drink large quantities of the infuſion of this vegetable, are ſo far from being remarkable for the number of their children, that I have been well informed, two births to a marriage is the common proportion in Holland *(d)*.

IT muſt be acknowledged, however, that warm infuſions of tea, by relaxing and augmenting the ſenſibility of the fibres, which in cold climates, and in hard labouring people, are uſually too rigid and torpid, may promote the increaſe of the human ſpecies. But the obſervation is true only under certain limitations; for the ſame cauſe, by debilitating the conſtitution beyond the due

(d) IN China, the women are ſo prolific, and the human ſpecies multiplies ſo faſt, that the lands, though ever ſo much cultivated, are ſcarcely ſufficient to ſupport the inhabitants. *Monteſquieu.*

medium,

medium, may operate in a contrary manner. Perhaps the general uſe of pepper, and of other ſpices, may increaſe the fertility of mankind.

But I ſhall ſuſpend my conjectures for the preſent. A variety of cauſes may counteract the operation of thoſe which I have enumerated; and a conſiderable number of facts muſt be adduced to aſcertain, whether the proportion of births to marriages be generally increaſed in countries advanced from poverty to wealth, by the introduction of trade, or the improvement of agriculture. The inſtance of Middleton, and of one or two places more which firſt occurred, and ſuggeſted the preceding obſervations, is oppoſed by others which have lately fallen under my notice. And I cannot cloſe this ſubject better, than by giving a view of all the facts, which I have collected on both ſides of the queſtion.

A Table *ſhewing the* Proportion *of* Births *to* Marriages *in different Places, and at different Periods of Time.*

MIDDLETON.

Year.	Marriages.	Chriſtenings.	Births to a Marriage.
From 1663 to 1672,	121	388	= $3\frac{1}{5}$+.
1763 to 1772,	330	1570	= $4\frac{3}{4}$.

WARRINGTON.

WARRINGTON.

Year.	Marriages.	Christenings.		Births to a Marriage.
From 1702 to 1722,	131	385	=	2.9.
1752 to 1772,	1549	5034	=	$3\frac{1}{4}$.

PENTRAETH PARISH, ANGLESEY*.

From 1740 to 1747,	32	100	=	$3\frac{1}{8}$.
1764 to 1771,	33	149	=	$4\frac{1}{2}$.

LLANDYFNAN PARISH, ANGLESEY*.

From 1750 to 1757,	28	111	=	3.9+.
1764 to 1771,	32	154	=	$4\frac{4}{5}$+.
1547 to 1554,	8	36	=	$4\frac{1}{2}$.
1620 to 1627,	20	44	=	$2\frac{1}{5}$.

LEVERPOOL.

From 1700 to 1710,	500	2127	=	$4\frac{1}{4}$.
1762 to 1771,	4812	10010	=	$2\frac{1}{12}$.

BOWDEN.

From 1653 to 1662,	136	573	=	$4\frac{1}{5}$+.
1763 to 1772,	369	1300	=	$3\frac{1}{2}$+.

MANCHESTER.

From 1763 to 1773,	4396	11052	=	$2\frac{1}{17}$.

* See Philosophical Transactions, vol. LXIII.

I HAVE

I HAVE lately received from the Rev. Mr. Archdeacon Blackburne, Rector of Richmond in Yorkſhire, the following account of his pariſh. From the year 1764 to 1773 incluſive, 452 males, and 376 females have been baptiſed; and 299 males, and 341 females have been buried. The marriages during this period have amounted to 200. In Richmond there are about ſix hundred houſes; but the Eaſter Book enumerates only 450 families; and Mr. Blackburne computes the number of inhabitants to be 2300. "We have no diſtempers," he ſays, "that can be "called endemial; and when fevers prevail in the "neighbourhood, few are affected by them in "this town. If any perſon brings an ague to "Richmond, he is generally freed from it in a "few days; though the village of Gilling, about "a mile and a half diſtant, which ſtands low, and "has a large pool of ſtagnant water adjoining to "it, is viſited with this complaint every ſpring "and autumn.

"THE air of Richmond ſeems to be peculiarly "unfavourable to conſumptive diſorders. Many "ſtrangers come hither, from different parts, in "the firſt ſtage of the *phthiſis pulmonalis*; but, "after thirty-five years experience, I may truly "ſay that not one has recovered; although the "utmoſt care and attention has been paid to "their reſpective caſes. The natives and con-"ſtant

"stant residents however are not subject to "distempers of the lungs, except when brought "on by intemperance. But rheumatic com-"plaints are very general, especially amongst "the senior part of the inhabitants. In small "corporation towns, like Richmond, numbers "are taken off by excessive drinking; but the "people here who live temperately, seldom die "earlier than in their eightieth year."

HAPPENING to pass through Sutton-Coldfield in Warwickshire, last summer, I was very much struck with the beauty and apparent healthfulness of its situation; and was desirous of knowing the duration of life which the inhabitants of it enjoy. The rector of the parish has, with great politeness and good nature, gratified my curiosity, as far as he is able, by furnishing me with an extract from the church register, and by referring me to the thirty-second volume of the Gentleman's Magazine, for the following authentic account of the place, drawn up, I suppose, by himself.

"SUTTON-COLDFIELD is almost full south of "Litchfield, at the distance of about eight "measured miles, by which it undoubtedly got "its name of Sutton, a contraction of South "town: A remarkably bleak and barren com-"mon, which lies directly west of it, just out "of the bounds of the parish, might probably "give it the additional denomination of Cold-

" field; the air being, upon that heath, as keen " and cold as in the Highlands of Scotland. " The pariſh is nearly oval in its figure; the " longeſt diameter ſeven miles, and the breadth " four. The face of it is agreeably diverſified " with gently riſing hills, and vallies of tolerably " fruitful meadows. It is bounded on the north " by Kenſton, on the weſt by Barr, on the ſouth " by Curdworth and Aſton near Birmingham, " and on the eaſt by Middleton: It contains " four hamlets, viz. Mancy, Hill, Little Sutton, " and Warmley. In the year 1630, there were " 298 houſes in the pariſh; in 1698 there were " 310; in 1721 the number was increaſed to " 360, which is nearly about the number at " preſent. I compute the inhabitants at 1800. " The regiſter begins in the year 1603. The " number of chriſtenings for the firſt 20 years " of the regiſter was 645; the burials during the " ſame period were 501. The number of " chriſtenings for the laſt 20 years (ending at " Chriſtmas 1761) was 747; the burials " 694 *(a)*."

It is curious to obſerve the almoſt exact proportion which the chriſtenings bear to the burials, in two very diſtant periods of time. But the like proportion ſeems to hold no longer. For

(a) Gentleman's Magazine for September 1762, p. 401.

from

from 1762 to 1772 the births have been 655, the deaths 445. The vicinity of Birmingham, and the amazing extenſion of its manufactures, will account for this change; which ſeems to have ariſen from the recruits annually drawn from Sutton-Coldfield, as well as from every other adjacent place. If the number of inhabitants in this town be rightly computed, the yearly mortality amongſt them is only as 1 to 51; and every houſe, at a medium, contains five perſons.

It appears by the obſervations lately communicated to me by the Rev. Doctor Tucker, that the number of females baptized at the pariſh church of St. Stephen's in Briſtol, from 1754 to 1774, has exceeded the number of males baptized during the ſame period of time; and that the like remark has been made in ſome other pariſhes of the ſame city. From theſe facts the learned Dean concludes, that Dr. Derham's calculation, which ſuppoſes the proportion of male to female births to be as 14 to 13, may probably be erroneous; and he expreſſes his earneſt wiſh, that further inquiry may be made into a ſubject of ſo much importance. The following table will ſhew the reſult of the few obſervations which I have collected.

A COMPARATIVE VIEW *of the* NUMBER *of* MALES *and* FEMALES, BAPTIZED *in different Places.*

Places.	Males.	Females.
Diſhley, 11 years -	149	145
St. Stephen's Pariſh, Briſtol, 20 years - -	591	607
Taxal, 16 years - -	204	230
Richmond, 10 years -	452	376
Middleton, 10 years -	200	188
Bowden, 10 years -	663	639
Middlewich, 5 years -	229	242
Chapel in le Frith, 10 years	451	332
Warrington, 1 year -	175	181
Collegiate Church in Mancheſter, 7 years -	3215	3024
Royton, 10 years -	134	120
Cheſter, 2 years -	408	415
Total	6871	6499

FROM this table it appears, that the proportion of males to females baptized is nearly as 12 to 11; but the ſucceeding ones ſhew, that the number of females alive conſiderably exceeds the number of males, in a variety of places; and that the widows are almoſt double the number of widowers.

A COMPARATIVE

A COMPARATIVE VIEW *of the* NUMBER *of* MALES *and* FEMALES *in different Places.*

Places.	Males.	Females.
Manchefter -	10548	11933
Salford - -	2248	2517
Townfhips of ditto	947	958
Parifh of Manchefter	6942	6844
Bolton - -	2159	2392
Little Bolton -	361	410
Monton - -	196	190
Hale - -	140	136
Horwich - -	149	156
Darwen - -	900	950
Cockey - -	320	391
Chowbent - -	554	606
Ackworth - -	340	388
Eaftham - -	451	461
Chinley - -	181	168
Brownfide -	40	47
Bugfworth -	80	95
Afhton under line	1406	1453
Parifh of ditto -	2584	2513
Tattenhall Parifh	382	399
Waverton Parifh	310	332
Total	31238	33339

A COMPARATIVE VIEW *of the* NUMBER *of* WIDOWERS *and* WIDOWS, *in different Places.*

Places.	Widowers.	Widows.
Mancheſter - -	432	1064
Salford - - -	89	149
Townſhip of ditto -	21	42
Pariſh of Mancheſter -	232	315
Monton - - -	14	13
Hale - - -	8	12
Horwich - - -	9	8
Darwen - - -	30	48
Cockey - - -	10	27
Chowbent - -	26	43
Chinley, Brownſide, and Bugſworth - -	15	18
Aſhton under line -	50	81
Pariſh of ditto - -	67	95
Total	1003	1915

LET no arguments in favour of polygamy be drawn from theſe tables! The practice is brutal; deſtructive to friendſhip and moral ſentiment; inconſiſtent with one great end of marriage, the education of children; and ſubverſive of the natural rights of more than half of the ſpecies.

- - - Higher

- - - - - Higher of the genial bed by far,
And with myſterious reverence I deem.

MILTON.

Nor is this tyranny of man over the weaker, but more amiable ſex, favourable to population. For notwithſtanding the number of females in the world may conſiderably exceed the number of males, yet there are more men capable of propagating their ſpecies, than women capable of bearing children. This painful office gradually becomes more dangerous, and leſs frequent, as the rigidneſs of the fibres increaſes; and ceaſes entirely at the age of fifty. The fatality of it is thus wiſely obviated, and the comforts of declining life are not interrupted by the arduous toil of nurſing. An inſtitution therefore which confines in ſervile bondage to one uſurper, many females in the prime of youth, muſt leave numbers deſtitute of the means which nature has pointed out, for perpetuating and increaſing the race of mankind. And it is a fact well known, that Armenia, in which a plurality of wives is not allowed, abounds more with inhabitants than any other province of the Turkiſh Empire.

JUNE 5, 1774.

P. S. SINCE the preceding paper was written, the Rev. Mr. Craddock has favoured me with a ſurvey of the town and pariſh of Aſhton under line, diſtant about eight miles from Mancheſter; and, alſo, with an account of the burials and chriſtenings, during the laſt eleven years. The inhabitants of this place conſiſt of manufacturers and farmers.

An ENUMERATION *of the* INHABITANTS *of the Town and Pariſh of* ASHTON UNDER LINE, *made in* 1775.

	Town.	Pariſh.
Inhabitants -	2859	5097
Houſes - -	553	941
Families - -	599	971
Males - -	1406	2584
Females - -	1453	2513
Married - -	982	1679
Widowers - -	50	67
Widows - -	81	95
Under five years of age	509	896
From five to ten	396	764
ten to twenty	541	1011
twenty to fifty	1044	1882
fifty to ſeventy	307	471
ſeventy to ninety	62	73

An

An Account of the BURIALS *and* CHRISTENINGS *in the Parish of* ASHTON UNDER LINE, *during the last eleven Years.*

BURIALS.

		Males unmarried.	Females Do.	Husbands.	Wives.	Widowers.	Widows.
1765	159	60	51	10	17	13	8
1766	187	42	54	34	24	7	26
1767	159	44	45	23	21	9	17
1768	197	69	60	18	25	1	24
1769	206	79	75	16	12	9	15
1770	167	54	46	29	7	20	11
1771	178	67	43	26	23	8	11
1772	250	97	71	16	35	10	21
1773	157	48	50	18	23	6	12
1774	152	38	46	21	24	10	13
1775	241	92	96	15	20	8	10
	2053	690	637	226	231	101	168

CHRISTENINGS.

	Males.	Females.
1765	121	114
1766	97	123
1767	116	111
1768	122	108
1769	157	137

1770

	Males.	Females.
1770	139	142
1771	133	143
1772	168	141
1773	174	131
1774	137	146
1775	168	164
	1532	1460

THE Reverend Dr. Peploe, Chancellor of the dioceſe of Cheſter, has honoured me with the following account of the pariſhes of Waverton and Tattenhall, both in the neighbourhood of Cheſter. The inhabitants are farmers and labourers.

An ENUMERATION *of the* INHABITANTS *of* TATTENHALL, *made in Auguſt* 1774, *by the Reverend* BRICE STORR, *Curate.*

Inhabited houſes - - -	148.
Uninhabited ditto - - -	2.
Heads of families - - -	176.
Aged above fifteen years - -	462.
Men and boys - - -	382.
Women and girls - - -	399.

CHRISTENINGS.

	CHRISTENINGS.	BURIALS.
1764	28	8
1765	21	9
1766	19	12
1767	29	11
1768	28	16
1769	24	15
1770	37	15
1771	30	9
1772	26	15
1773	38	20
	280	130

An ENUMERATION *of the* INHABITANTS *of* WAVERTON, *made in August* 1774, *by the Reverend Mr.* BISSELL, *Minister of the Parish.*

Inhabited houses	109
Uninhabited ditto	2
Heads of families	116
Aged above fourteen years	406
Men and boys	310
Women and girls	332

	CHRISTENINGS.	BURIALS.
1764	19	10
1765	26	2
1766	17	7
1767	18	10

	CHRISTENINGS.	BURIALS.
1768	22	10
1769	17	7
1770	20	8
1771	23	9
1772	18	12
1773	13	9
	193	84

EXTRACT *of a* LETTER *from the Reverend Mr.* BISSELL, *of* WAVERTON *near* CHESTER.

At the beginning of the year 1775, the pariſh of Waverton near Cheſter, contained

Inhabited Houſes.	Families.	Males.	Females.	Inhabitants.
111.	116.	310.	332.	642.

From Jan. 1ſt to Dec. 31ſt 1775 incluſive there were

CHRISTENINGS.		BURIALS.	
Males	14	Males	6
Females	8	Females	6
	22		12

BURIALS IN 1775.

Days.	Sex.	Age.	Diſeaſes.
Jan. 20,	A Woman	77 Years	Aſthma.
Jan. 31,	A Girl	9 Weeks	Convulſions.
Feb. 9,	A Woman	67 Years	Dropſy.
March 6,	A Woman	87 Years	Decay of Age, and an Ulcer in the Axilla.

April

Days.	Sex.	Age.	Diseases.
April 3,	A Woman	65 Years	Putrid Fever.
April 9,	A Man	45 Years	Uncertain.
April 11,	A Man	63 Years	Dropsy.
June 18,	A Woman	40 Years	Consumption.
July 6,	A Boy	14 Months	Small Pox with hot Regimen.
Aug. 14,	A Boy	4 Years	Small Pox and Worms.
Nov. 11,	A Man	65 Years	Gout and Dropsy in consequence of hard drinking.
Nov. 26,	A Man	68 Years	Dropsy.

In the valuable work which I have so often quoted, Dr. Price has advanced many arguments to shew the declining state of population in this kingdom. The growth of large towns, the prevalence of vice and luxury, the discouragements to marriage, the destruction of cottages, and various other causes, have the most unfavourable influence on the increase of mankind. But it is to be hoped, that these evils do not generally prevail, and that even some good may arise from them to check their baneful effects. Certain it is, that in this part of England the inhabitants multiply with great rapidity: And though the increase may be chiefly owing to recruits drawn from other counties, yet the flourishing state of our manufactures cannot fail to promote population, by affording plentiful means

means of ſubſiſtence to the poor. The Biſhop of Cheſter (Dr. Markham) informs me, that in various pariſh regiſters which he has conſulted, the births have progreſſively become more numerous from generation to generation. At Broxley in Kent, where his Lordſhip was Vicar, he divided the times, from the commencement of the reign of Queen Elizabeth, into periods of twenty-one years; and found, that the number of births in the firſt period was 310, and in the laſt 525. The increaſe was gradual through the whole time.

APPENDIX

TO THE FOREGOING OBSERVATIONS.

THE following view of the progreſs of population, in Mancheſter, from 1758 to 1777, incluſive, divided into periods of five years, was annexed to the yearly bill of mortality, A.D. 1778.

	Average Number of Deaths including Diſſenters.	Number of Inhabitants eſtimated by ſuppoſing the Deaths to be 1 in 28,4.	Progreſſive Increaſe.
From 1758 to 1762	751	21,328	——.
1763 to 1767	869	24,680	3,352.
1768 to 1772	958	27,246	2,566.
1773 to 1777	1010	28,684	1,438.

DURING

During the laſt-mentioned period, viz. from 1773 to 1777, 719 houſes were built in Mancheſter and Salford. At the cloſe of 1777, 151 of theſe were uninhabited.

By a ſurvey, completed in December, 1783, of the townſhips of Mancheſter and Salford, the number of houſes was found be 6195; which number multiplied, as formerly, by 6$\frac{1}{3}$ would make the inhabitants to have then amounted to 39,235. But it is probable, that the proportion of 6$\frac{1}{3}$ to a houſe, is leſs than the truth, at a period when the reſtoration of peace produced a ſudden influx of people. And the increaſe of population has been ſince ſo great, that the enumeration at Chriſtmas, 1788, ſtood as follows:

	Houſes.	Families.	Perſons.
Townſhip of Mancheſter,	5916	8570	42821.
Townſhip of Salford, about,	1260	——	——

In Salford, the houſes being generally ſmaller than in Mancheſter, Mr. Wharmby, the ſurveyor to whom I am indebted for this account, is of opinion, that ſix perſons may be reckoned to each dwelling. The whole number of inhabitants, therefore, in the two townſhips, exceeds 50,000.

The rapid growth of Mancheſter admits of an eaſy and ſatisfactory explanation, from the aſtoniſhing and ſudden increaſe of the cotton manufactory, of which it may be deemed the great

great *emporium*. Not more than twenty years ſince, it is ſaid, the whole annual return of this trade in Great Britain amounted only to £200,000: Whereas, at this time, the groſs produce of raw materials and labour is eſtimated at more than ſeven millions ſterling. And it is calculated, that one hundred and fifty-nine thouſand men, ninety thouſand women, and a hundred and one thouſand children are employed in the different ſtages of the manufacture *(b)*.

I HAVE mentioned an obſervation, communicated by Dr. Tucker, that the number of females baptized at the pariſh church of St. Stephen's, in Briſtol, from 1754 to 1774, exceeded the number of males baptized during the ſame period of time; and that, from hence, the learned Dean ſuſpected Dr. Derham's calculation to be erroneous, which makes the proportion of male to female births to be as 14 to 13. From the facts which I collected, the proportion appeared to be nearly as 12 to 11: But Dr. Price, from a much larger induction, has now fully ſhewn, that it is as 20 to 19 *(c)*.

(b) See a Pamphlet entitled, an Important Criſis in the Callico and Muſlin Manufactory. 1788.

(c) Reverſionary Payments, vol. II. fourth edit. p. 16. Appendix.

It has been evinced, by a great variety of regiſters, that the mortality of males exceeds that of females, in almoſt every period of life; but eſpecially in the earlieſt ſtages of it, nearly one half more of the former than of the latter being ſtill born; and, that the exceſs prevails moſt in great towns, and under other circumſtances, which are unfavourable to health. Dr. Clarke, phyſician to the Lying-in Hoſpital at Dublin, has elucidated this intricate ſubject, in a paper read before the Royal Society, March 30, 1786. Male fœtuſes, being larger, require more nutrition than female fœtuſes, during geſtation; and are more liable to injury at the time of birth. Debility, therefore, in either parent, from whatever ſource it may ariſe, muſt affect that ſex the moſt, both before and after delivery, which not only requires the largeſt and ſtrongeſt *ſtamina*, but is put to the ſevereſt trials, both in delivery and in after-life.

Among the cauſes which increaſe the proportion of human mortality, in large towns, muſt be reckoned the more ready communication and greater malignity of contagious diſtempers. In June 1783, I received the following information from Richard Townley, Eſq. of Belfield, near Rochdale, a very reſpectable and intelligent juſtice of the peace. I ſhall deliver it in his own words. "It is unneceſſary "to make any apology for ſending you an "account of the ravages, which that dreadful "diſorder, the ſmall-pox, made in the town "of Rochdale, within the ſpace of a few months, "laſt winter, compared with the ſtate of thoſe "children, who happened to be infected with "the ſame loathſome malady, in two villages "nearly adjoining to my houſe, during the "ſame period of time. The account is very "accurate, being taken by the conſtables, "who went from houſe to houſe; and it "is found to agree with the pariſh regiſter. "The latter table is delivered from my own "perſonal knowledge."

	No. Ill.	Dead.	Recovered.
Part of Huddersfield townſhip, within Rochdale,	141	40	101
Spotland townſhip, -	108	30	78
Caſtleton ditto, -	160	32	128
	409	102	307
In the village of Belfield,	20	0	20
Ditto Newbold,	19	1	18
	39	1	38

Dr. Smith, in the Wealth of Nations, obſerves, that it is not uncommon, in the Highlands

lands of Scotland, for a woman to have only two ſurviving children of twenty whom ſhe has brought into the world. But a life of rural labour, in a tolerably genial climate, without extreme penury, is favourable to population. At Dunmow in Eſſex, we are informed, the pariſh contains 262 poor families, who have 460 children. There are alſo 116 families of the ranks above them, who have only 120 children, which is little more than half the former proportion. The *ratio* of deaths, during the laſt five years, has been, of the poor children 1 in 45½; of thoſe in a higher ſtation 1 in 37½ *(d)*.

(d) See Howlett on the Increaſe of the Poor. 1788 p. 102.

ESSAY II.

ON THE

SMALL-POX AND MEASLES(*a*).

TABLES *ſhewing the* NUMBER *of* DEATHS *occaſioned by the* SMALL-POX, *in the ſeveral Periods of Life, and different Seaſons of the Year, together with its* COMPARATIVE FATALITY *to* MALES *and* FEMALES; *extracted from the Regiſter of the Collegiate or Pariſh Church in* MANCHESTER, *and from other* BILLS *of* MORTALITY.

ACCURATE and comprehenſive bills of mortality furniſh a variety of the moſt curious and important obſervations; and it is to be lamented that they are not univerſally adopted. The general uſes to which they may be applied, have been fully pointed out; and a plan for the eſtabliſhment of them has been propoſed to the conſideration and correction of the public (*b*). It is one part of this plan, that the regiſter of burials ſhall not only contain

(*a*) Inſerted in the London Medical Obſervations and Inquiries, vol. V. p. 270. (*b*) See vol. I. p. 428.

contain a lift of the difeafes of which all die, but alfo exprefs particularly the numbers dying of each difeafe, *in the feveral divifions of life, and different feafons of the year.* The following tables will illuftrate the advantages, which may be derived from this improvement.

An Account of DEATHS *by the* SMALL-POX, *during* SIX YEARS, *viz. from* 1768 *to* 1774; *collected from the Regifter of the Collegiate Church at* MANCHESTER.

TABLE I.

Ages.	Males.	Fe-males.	Annual Deaths by the Small-Pox.		Deaths by all Difeafes.
From Birth to 3 Months.	2.	2.	A. D.		
From 3 Months to 6 Months	9.	8.	1769.	74.	549.
			1770.	41.	689.
- - - - - to 1 Year	51.	68.	1771.	182.	678.
2.	103.	113.	1772.	66.	608.
3.	55.	55.	1773.	139.	648.
4.	33.	26.	1774.	87.	635.
5.	18.	16.			
10.	17.	12.			
20.	1.	0.			
30.	0.	0.			
Total	289.	300.		589.*	3807.

I. THIS

* THIS account of the annual deaths by the fmall-pox from 1768 to 1774, differs from the printed bills of mor-

I. This table is formed from a very accurate regifter, and affords a ftriking view of the difparity in the ravages of the fmall-pox, at different periods of life. The proportion of deaths under the age of three months is extremely fmall; and I think we may conclude, that this diftemper rarely occurs in the early part of infancy. For children in that tender feafon are neither in the way of infection, nor does experience fhew that they are much difpofed to receive it. Dr. Monro informs us, that of twelve infants, inoculated within a fortnight, after their birth, not one had the variolous eruption *(c)*. In the fecond ftage of infancy, the fatality of the fmall-pox is fomewhat increafed; but the advancement proceeds afterwards with amazing rapidity. For, during the eighteen months which next fucceed, the number of deaths amounts to 335; which is more than one half of all that occur through the remainder of life. At this period, therefore, we may prefume that the body is peculiarly liable to the difeafe; and the violence and malignity of it are aggravated by the breed-

tality; which make the number amount to 586, and not to 589. But it has been extracted from the church regifter with a degree of care and attention not ufually beftowed upon the printed bills; and the accuracy of it may, I believe, be relied upon.

(c) Monro on Inoculation, p. 25.

ing

ing of teeth, and by the general irritability of the nervous ſyſtem. But the firſt dentition is uſually completed before the end of the third year; at which time the ſmall-pox appears, by the table, to become conſiderably leſs mortal. And its declenſion is not leſs rapid than its progreſs, as the conſtitution improves in vigour, and as thoſe decreaſe in number who are liable to its attack.

In the year 1773, the ſmall-pox raged with great violence in the town of Warrington; and I have procured from my friend Mr. John Aikin, an exact account of the number and ages of thoſe who died of it. This account coincides with the foregoing table, and confirms many of the concluſions which are deducible from it.

DEATHS BY THE SMALL-POX AT WARRINGTON IN 1773.

TABLE II.

Ages.					Numbers.
Under	1	Month			0.
From	1	to	3	Months	4.
	3	--	6	- - -	6.
	6	--	12	- - -	39.
From	1	to	2	Years	84.
	2	--	3	- - -	33.
	3	--	4	- - -	18.
	4	--	5	- - -	15.

Ages.				Numbers.
From 5	to	6	Years	4.
6	--	7	---	2.
7	--	8	---	2.
8	--	9	---	4.
None above.			Total	211.

II. THE ſmall-pox, by table I. appears to have been more fatal to female than to male children, and the difference is conſiderable under the age of two years. At Warrington, two thirds of all who died of this diſeaſe in 1773 were females. Theſe facts are ſomewhat extraordinary; as it has been fully evinced by a variety of obſervations, that the life of males is much more frail than that of females *(d)*, and particularly in the period of infancy *(e)*. They alſo contradict the following remark of Baron Van Swieten: *Cum autem muliebre Corpus mollius et laxius ſit corpore virili, hinc, cæteris paribus, & in his mitior eſſe ſolet hic morbus.*

Comment. vol. V. p. 16.

III. THE comparative mortality of the ſmall-pox at Mancheſter, Warrington, and Chowbent, in the different ſeaſons of the year, may be eſtimated by the following table.

(d) SEE Dr. Price's Treatiſe on Reverſionary Payments, *paſſim*; alſo the preceding Obſervations on the State of Population in Mancheſter, and other adjacent Places.

(e) Ibid.

TABLE

TABLE III.

Months.	Manchester, From 1768 to 1774.	Warrington, 1773.	Chowbent, From 1767 to 1773	Total.
January, February, March,	160.	21.	17.	198.
April, May, June,	137.	135.	7.	279.
July, Auguſt, September,	147.	51.	2.	200.
October, November, December.	145.	4.	1.	150.

Sydenham has obſerved, that the ſmall-pox, when it is mild and regular, uſually commences about the vernal equinox, in thoſe years in which it is epidemic; but that it begins earlier when it is of an irregular and more dangerous kind. No one can doubt, that variations in the moiſture, dryneſs, temperature, and other qualities of the air, muſt influence a diſeaſe, which is always of an inflammatory, and often, in its laſt ſtages, of a putrid nature. But the progreſs of it cannot be regulated by the ſeaſons, becauſe it is derived from contagion; the communication of which frequently depends upon accident, is confined to no period of time, and is varied by its degrees of of malignity. During the late viſitation of the ſmall-pox at Warrington, the ſtate of the atmoſphere went through all poſſible changes, but with no perceptible difference in the circumſtances of the diſeaſe *(f)*.

IV. During the period of time included in the firſt table, the ſmall-pox was twice epidemical in Mancheſter; and the deaths by it amount nearly to one ſixth and a half of thoſe occaſioned by all other diſeaſes. But it may be proper to remark, that the poor of this town are chiefly buried at the collegiate church; and this diſtemper proves much more fatal to them than to perſons of better rank, from their want of cleanlineſs, and their prejudice in favour of a hot regimen. In London, from 1762 to 1772, the average proportion of deaths by the ſmall-pox is 109 in 1000, or about a ninth of the whole. And at Ackworth, a country pariſh near Ferrybridge in Yorkſhire, the proportion during twenty years, viz. from 1747 to 1767, is as 1 to 19; two hundred and ſixty-three perſons having been buried, fourteen of whom died of the ſmall-pox. Were ſuch accounts to be collected from different places, and at different periods of time, it is probable, that farther variations in the fata-

(f) See Philoſophical Tranſactions, vol. LXIV. p. 439.

lity of this diſeaſe would be diſcovered *(g)*. But from its leaſt deſtructive ravages we may derive arguments of ſufficient force, in favour of inoculation. And the two firſt tables may perhaps furniſh ſome uſeful information, concerning the particular ſeaſon of life in which this practice will be moſt expedient, and attended with the greateſt proſpect of ſucceſs.

(g) BARON Van Swieten has given the following remarkable account of the proportion of deaths by the ſmall-pox, in ſeveral ſchools and hoſpitals at Vienna. *Ratione ſubducta, patet, quod numerus omnium, qui in his locis variolis decubuerunt, ſit* 355, *et quod ex hoc numero ſeptem mortui fuerint. Adeoq; proportio mortuorum ad numerum ſanatorum eſt ut* 1. *ad* 50. *circiter. Si autem de hoc mortuorum numero detraherentur tres aegri, quorum mors ſolis variolis adſcribi nequit, tunc certe proportio mortuorum ad ſanatos foret ut* 1. *ad* 89. *circiter.*

Van Swieten. Comment. vol. V. p. 145.

MR. BEW, an ingenious apothecary in Mancheſter, informs me, that he attended ſeventy patients the laſt year (1774) under the natural ſmall-pox, of which number only two died. They were chiefly children above the age of two years; and the cool regimen was ſtrictly purſued in the treatment of them.

In the ſecondary fever of the ſmall-pox, I have known a *warm bath*, prepared of a decoction of chamomile leaves and flowers, with a proper quantity of butter-milk added to it, produce the happieſt effects. It cleanſes the ſkin from the putrid *ſordes* which covers it; ſoftens the puſtules; opens the pores; promotes perſpiration; and proves highly refreſhing to the patient.

V. If we regard only the ſtate of the body, the fitteſt period for the ingraftment of the ſmall-pox ſeems to be between the age of two and four in healthy children, and of three and ſix in thoſe who are tender and delicate. The powers of nature are then ſufficiently vigorous; perſpiration is free and copious; the irritability of the body is diminiſhed; the viſcera are ſound and unobſtructed; the mind, though active and lively, is not diſturbed by violent emotions; the teguments are properly extenuated; and the fibres are neither too tenſe nor too lax for the variolous eruption. To theſe important advantages may be added, that at this age the child is both a proper ſubject for preparatory medicines, and for ſuch as may be deemed neceſſary during the courſe of the diſtemper. But other conſiderations, beſides the ſtate of the conſtitution, demand our attention. The riſque of receiving the natural ſmall-pox by infection appears to be very great during the ſecond year of life; and the fatality of the diſeaſe at this period is highly alarming. To avert ſuch impending danger, the inoculation of healthy and vigorous children, at the *age of two or three months*, ſeems to be adviſeable, eſpecially in large towns. An earlier period might complicate the ſmall-pox with the jaundice, thruſh, gripes, diarrhœa, and other diſorders incident to the firſt ſtage of infancy; and a later ſeaſon may ſuperadd

ſuperadd the fever, convulſions, and other ſymptoms of dentition. But I have enlarged upon this ſubject in the former volume, to which I refer the reader *(b)*.

My friend Dr. Haygarth, to whom I communicated the preceding *Tables of the comparative mortality of the ſmall-pox, &c.* has adopted the plan, and purſued the ſame inquiry at Cheſter. His ſtatement will ſhew how exactly our obſervations agree.

CHESTER, 1774.

Total of deaths by the ſmall-pox, - 202.
Deaths by the ſmall-pox under 1 year old, 51.

(b) See vol. I. p. 230.

In a letter from the Hon. and Rev. Mr. Stuart, rector of Luton in Bedfordſhire, to Sir William Fordyce, dated March 1, 1788, it is ſaid, that of 1215 patients inoculated in that pariſh, only five died, and thoſe at the following ages.

Perſons.	Ages.		
1	9	weeks old,	thruſh.
1	7	ditto.	
1	12	ditto.	
1	16	ditto.	of a fit.
1	5	ditto.	

viz.

viz.		Males.	Females.
Under	1 month,	0.	0.
Between	1 and 2 months,	1.	1.
	2 and 3,	1.	0.
	3 and 6,	2.	2.
	6 and 9,	12.	10.
	9 and 12,	6.	16.
	Total	22.	29.

TABLES *of the* COMPARATIVE MORTALITY *of the* MEASLES *from* 1768 *to* 1774, *collected from the Register of the Collegiate Church in* MANCHESTER.

T A B L E I.

Ages.	Males.	Females.	Seasons.	Total of Deaths by all Diseases, during 6 Years.
From Birth to 3 Months	1.	1.	Jan. Feb. March } 17.	
From 3 Months to 6 Months	3.	0.		
1 Year	6.	4.	April May June } 51.	
2.	17.	14.		
3.	17.	8.		
4.	4.	3.	July Aug. Sep. } 16.	
5.	2.	7.		
10.	0.	2.		
20.	0.	1.	Oct. Nov. Dec. } 7.	
30.	0.	1.		
Total	50.	41.	91*.	3807.

THIS

* THIS, like the first table of the small-pox, differs in the total of deaths by the measles, from the printed bills of mortality.

THIS table requires no comments. The proportional mortality of the meaſles, in the ſeveral periods of life, and various ſeaſons of the year, is obvious at the firſt view. It is equally evident alſo, that this diſeaſe differs from the ſmall-pox, in being much more fatal to males than to females.

DURING the ſpring and ſummer months of the year 1774, the meaſles were epidemical in Mancheſter, and proved fatal to a conſiderable number of children. They were of the regular kind, ſo well deſcribed by Sydenham; but it was not unuſual for violent peripneumonic ſymptoms to occur, five, ſix, or even eight days after the diſappearance of the eruption. Under theſe circumſtances venæſection, bliſters, and the Seneka root were found to be very efficacious remedies.

tality. I have therefore deſired Mr. Holme, one of the clerks of the collegiate church, a very intelligent man and a good arithmetician, to reviſe the church regiſter; and after the moſt careful inſpection, he aſſures me, that the numbers in both tables are perfectly accurate. He ſays, "The printed "bills of mortality are exact as to the number of deaths, "and the diviſion of males and females; but when the diſ-"orders are counted over, and the general amount is taken, "there is often a miſtake in the ſum total. And, as it is "a great trouble and difficulty to diſcover wherein the "error lies, and as few perſons pay any regard to this part "of the bills, it is common to add the number deficient to "ſome of the diſorders, ſo as to make the whole agree."

I preſcribed

I prescribed the Peruvian bark with great success to many of my patients under the measles, combining it with demulcents, and the saline mixture; and premising venæsection when the signs of inflammation were urgent. The practice of giving the bark in this disease was first introduced by Dr. Cameron, a very eminent physician at Worcester. He observes that it prevents the recession of the morbid acrimony, and continues the efflorescence on the skin, sometimes so long as the twelfth day *(i)*. By this salutary operation, the cough and other inflammatory symptoms are in a great measure obviated; and the patient is freed from all danger of a peripneumony, the fatality of which Sydenham describes in such strong terms. It is many years since I first adopted the method of cure recommended by Dr. Cameron; and experience has afforded me the fullest conviction of its safety and efficacy, in all ordinary cases. During the late epidemic, not a single instance occurred to me of the peripneumony succeeding the measles, when the bark had been employed. But my assistance was desired in the last stage of fifteen unfortunate cases of this kind, in which the common antiphlogistic and pectoral course had been pursued.

(i) Medical Museum, vol. I. No. 37, p. 281.

The meafles, when violent in degree, or ill treated, frequently lay the foundation of hectic fevers, or pulmonary confumptions. For as the infection is moft probably conveyed by infpiration, the lungs become inflamed, a cough enfues, tubercles or a vomica are formed, and the patient finks under a lingering, painful, and incurable difeafe. To obviate thefe evils, inoculation was propofed about fifteen years ago, and practifed, in feveral inftances, with confiderable fuccefs by Dr. Home. The forenefs of the eyes was mitigated by it, the cough abated, and the fever rendered lefs fevere. His method of communicating the infection was by applying, to an incifion in each arm, cotton moiftened with the blood of a patient labouring under the meafles *(k)*. But the morbillous matter has fince been ingrafted by means of lint, wet with the tears, which flow from the eyes in the firft ftage of this diforder. For thefe laudable endeavours to extend the benefits of inoculation, the public is highly indebted to Dr. Home; and it is to be lamented, that fo little attention has been paid to this valuable improvement of the healing art.

The following table fhews the annual medium of deaths by the fmall-pox and meafles, from 1754 to 1774, compared with the deaths under

(k) Home's Medical Facts and Experiments.

two years of age by all diſeaſes, and with the general amount of births and deaths during the ſame period of time. It is collected from the printed bills of mortality, publiſhed yearly at Mancheſter.

TABLE II.

Years.	Small-Pox.	Meaſles.	Under 2 Years of Age.	Total of Deaths.	Births.
From 1754 to 1758	64.	21.	209.	651.	678.
to 1764*.	95.	10.6.	213.	639.	731.
to 1769.	98.	9.6.	229.	659.	827.
to 1774.	102.	21.6.	242.	651.	1002.
Total	359.	62.8.	893.	2600.	3238.

This table comprehends ſo long a term of years, that the inferences which it affords would be no leſs indubitable than important, if we could entirely rely upon the accuracy of the *printed bills of mortality*. I apprehend, however, the errors of theſe bills are not conſiderable;

* I am not in poſſeſſion of the bill of mortality for the year 1760; which is therefore omitted in this table.

and

and that the following conclusions, with respect to Manchester, may be admitted as approaching very near to TRUTH.

I. ONE in *nine*, of all whose births are registered at baptism, dies of the SMALL-POX; and nearly *one* in *fifty-two* of the MEASLES. It should be observed, that the births considerably exceed the burials at Manchester.

II. THE deaths by the MEASLES are to the deaths by the SMALL-POX, as *one* to *five* and *eight tenths*.

III. THE number dying under two YEARS OF AGE, of all diseases, is to the number baptized, as *one* to *three* and *six tenths*.

IV. THE number dying under two YEARS OF AGE is to the total number of deaths, as *one* to *two* and *nine tenths*.

V. THE deaths by the SMALL-POX are to the deaths by all diseases, nearly as *one* to *seven* and *a quarter*.

VI. NEARLY *three fifths* of those who are carried off by the SMALL-POX die under the age of two years (see table I. of the small-pox); and *one* in *four* of all that die under two years of age fall victims to this disease.

VII. HALF of the deaths occasioned by the MEASLES happen under two years of age; and the proportion which this number bears to the general deaths, under the ſame period, is nearly as *one* to *twenty-eight*.

Many other very important corollaries may be deduced from this and the preceding tables; but I wiſh rather to excite, than to anticipate the inquiries of the intelligent reader.

Feb. 1, 1775.

ESSAY III.

AN ATTEMPT TO ACCOUNT FOR THE

DIFFERENT QUANTITIES OF RAIN,

WHICH FALL AT

DIFFERENT HEIGHTS OVER THE SAME SPOT OF GROUND (a).

IT is a reflection which may mortify pride and humble arrogance, but which ought certainly to animate the ſpirit of patient attention, and conſole us under the diſappointments of philoſophical purſuits, that many of the moſt intereſting laws of nature have remained undiſcovered, till ſome happy coincidence of circumſtances hath pointed them out to inquiry or obſervation. Thus, the energy of fire muſt have been known and felt from the creation of the world; but the regularity of its expanſile power, on different bodies, is a modern diſcovery, of uncertain date. And the

(a) Inſerted in Dr. Hunter's Georgical Eſſays, p. 257, 8vo. edit.

 real

real nature of this ſubtile element, which pervades and actuates all matter, and is continually perceptible to our ſenſes, is yet but imperfectly explored. The ancients were acquainted with the magnifying power of *denſe mediums*; and Seneca has noticed, that ſmall letters appear larger and brighter when viewed through a glaſs globe filled with water. He has remarked, alſo, that apples are more beautiful, when ſwimming in ſuch a veſſel. But theſe obſervations, which muſt have been made by numberleſs ſpectators, in a long ſucceſſion of years, were regarded as ſolitary facts; and it was not till the thirteenth century, that ſpectacles were conſtructed, in conſequence, probably, of the experiments made by the Arabian philoſopher Alhazen, and our juſtly celebrated countryman Roger Bacon. Yet though magnifying glaſſes came then into general uſe, and muſt have been daily handled by artiſts and others, three hundred years elapſed before it occurred to any one to put them together, ſo as to form a teleſcope. The collection of watery vapours in the air, the figures of clouds, and the deſcent of rain, could paſs, in no age, unnoticed by mankind, and have long been the ſubjects of attentive inveſtigation. Yet it is a very recent diſcovery, which we owe to the ſagacity of a moſt ingenious phyſician and philoſopher, that a manifeſt difference ſubſiſts in the quantity of rain which

which falls, at different heights, over the ſame ſpot of ground.

IN the laſt volume of the Philoſophical Tranſactions, (vol. LIX.) ſome experiments are related, by which it appears, that there fell below the top of a houſe, above a fifth part more rain, than what fell in the ſame ſpace above the top of the ſame houſe; and that there fell upon Weſtminſter Abbey, not above one half of what was found to fall in the ſame ſpace, below the tops of the houſes *(b)*. Theſe obſervations, however new

(b) I AM informed by an ingenious correſpondent at Bath, that ſimilar experiments have been made in that place, with the ſame reſult; and a friend at Leverpool, on whoſe judgment and accuracy I can rely with confidence, has lately favoured me with the following account, dated March 14th, 1771, "During the late rains, I repeated doctor "Heberden's experiment: The upper veſſel received thirteen "ounces and a half of rain, the lower veſſel twenty-ſeven "ounces. The difference of altitude was about ſixteen or "ſeventeen yards. The wind blew a briſk gale from the "South Eaſt.——I made the trial alſo during a fall of ſnow; "and in that, found the proportion as three to five." The following experiment, communicated to me by the ſame gentleman, varies a little in its reſult from the former, owing, perhaps, to a difference in the ſerenity of the air: For the wind has a more powerful effect on the deſcent of ſnow, than of rain, becauſe its ſpecific gravity is leſs. "March 27th, "1771, there was a continued fall of ſnow, from eight in the "morning till five in the afternoon. The air was ſtill; the "ſnow came down very thick, and in large flakes. During "the

new and ſingular, are too well authenticated to admit of the leaſt degree of doubt; and philoſophy ſhould be employed not in controverting a fact ſo fully aſcertained, but in furniſhing a rational and adequate cauſe of it.

DOCTOR HEBERDEN conjectures, that this phænomenon depends on ſome property of electricity, which he thinks remains hitherto unknown. To me it appears probable, that the common laws by which this power influences the aſcent and ſuſpenſion of vapours, are ſufficient to explain their precipitation in rain, and the lately diſcovered mode of its deſcent.

THE electrical fluid is ſtrongly attracted by water; and by deſtroying the coheſion between its particles, and repelling them from each other,

" the nine hours, which the ſnow continued to fall, the upper " veſſel received thirteen ounces, the lower veſſel twenty-ſix " ounces." In the years 1773 and 1774, the obſervations on the different quantities of rain, which fall at different heights, were repeatedly made at Leverpool. And it was almoſt uniformly found, that a veſſel, ſtanding on the ground in a ſpacious garden, received *double* the quantity of rain which fell into another veſſel, of equal dimenſions, placed near the ſame ſpot, but eighteen yards higher. At Middlewich, during part of the year 1774, the quantity of rain received at the top of the church ſteeple was 15,75 inches; and 19 inches in a garden, eighty feet below. The garden, it ſhould be remarked, was not contiguous to, although at no great diſtance from the church.

it becomes a powerful agent in evaporation. The waters of the ocean abound in this fire, and vapours raised from them float in the air, forming clouds, which retain their electricity till they meet with other bodies, either destitute of it, or containing it in a less proportion than themselves (c). This, in all probability, is frequently the case with those vapours or clouds which are produced by exhalations from the earth, from fresh water, and the perspiration of plants and trees; at least it is an undoubted fact, that some clouds (to use the language of this branch of philosophy) are electrified *positively*, and others *negatively*. No sooner does a communication take place, but the repulsion between the particles of water is diminished, those which have discharged part of their electricity are successively attracted by the contiguous ones which have not, and thus they press nearer together, become specifically heavier than the atmosphere, and descend in small drops, which, losing every instant more and more of the electric fire, coalesce, uniting into larger and larger drops, and consequently filling a space which is continually diminishing, as they approach nearer to the surface of the earth. This may be illustrated by electrifying the stream of a fountain, which

(c) Vide Franklin on Electricity.

will

will ſpread itſelf into the form of a bruſh by the mutual receſſion of the particles of water: But withdraw the ſupply of electric fire, and the fountain diſcharges itſelf in one continued current *(d)*. A pair of cork balls ſuſpended together by ſilken threads, when electrified recede from each other, and if the air be dry, return by degrees only to their natural poſition. Two feathers electrified will float in the atmoſphere, mutually repelling each other, when in a certain degree of contiguity, and gradually deſcending as they loſe that power, which by expanding their *plumulæ*, rendered them ſpecifically lighter than the air. But if one of them diſcharges ſuddenly the electric fire, it will inſtantly be attracted towards the other, and receive a freſh ſupply; when a repulſion (acting indeed at a much leſs diſtance than before) will again take place between them.

When two clouds, one replete with electric fire, the other deſtitute of it, come within the ſphere of each other's attraction, they will ruſh together, and the electrical fluid being diffuſed through a larger ſpace, the particles of water will unite, and form themſelves into drops of greater magnitude, and a heavy ſhower will be produced. Still however as the rain deſcends

(d) Vide Franklin on Electricity.

through

through an atmoſphere containing little electric fire, it will be continually communicating it, and the diſcharge being greateſt from the circumference of the cloud, becauſe the ſurface is there largeſt, the drops will be drawn nearer and nearer to each other, and, approaching towards one common centre, will gradually coaleſce in their paſſage. Doctor Franklin has related a moſt ingenious experiment, which elucidates the formation of rain as thus deſcribed.——Take two round pieces of paſteboard of two inches diameter; from the centre and circumference of each of them, ſuſpend, by fine ſilk threads eighteen inches long, ſeven ſmall balls of wood, or ſeven peas equal in bigneſs; ſo will the balls appending to each paſteboard, form equal equilateral triangles, one ball being in the centre, and ſix at equal diſtances from that and each other; and thus they repreſent particles of air. Dip both ſets in water, and, ſome adhering to each ball, they will repreſent air loaded. Dexterouſly electrify one ſet, and its balls will repel each other to a greater diſtance, enlarging the triangles. Could the water ſupported by the ſeven balls come into contact, it would form a drop or drops ſo heavy as to break the coheſion it had with the balls, and ſo fall. Let the two ſets then repreſent two clouds, the one a ſea cloud electrified, the other a land cloud; bring them

them within the ſphere of attraction, and they will draw towards each other, and you will ſee the ſeparated balls cloſe thus:—The firſt electrified ball that comes near an unelectrified ball, by attraction, joins it and gives it fire; inſtantly they ſeparate, and each flies to another ball of its own party, one to give, the other to receive fire; and ſo it proceeds through both ſets, but ſo quick as to be, in a manner, inſtantaneous. In their colliſion they ſhake off and drop their water, which repreſents rain. This experiment would better illuſtrate and confirm my *hypotheſis*, if a large number of balls were appended, at equal diſtances, to each paſteboard, ſo as to form ſeveral circles, having one common centre.

But it rarely happens, that a land cloud is equal in magnitude to one raiſed from the ſea; conſequently the rain produced by their union, will be proportionably lighter in the upper, and heavier in the lower regions of the atmoſphere, as the electric matter is more or leſs gradually diffuſed.

When an electrified cloud, without mixing with another cloud, or loſing part of its electric fire, becomes ſpecifically heavier than the atmoſphere, by cold, or ſome local change in the denſity of the air, it will deſcend at firſt perhaps in a miſt; but will form, as it approaches nearer to the earth,

earth, and is lefs replete with the electric fluid, a light fhower of rain.

Besides the clouds which float feparately in the higher regions of the atmofphere, the air contains a large quantity of water in the ftate both of folution and of diffufion; and dews, fogs, and fometimes even fhowers of rain, are probably produced by the precipitation of the water thus fufpended (c). Now the quantity of water which the air is capable of diffolving and fufpending, is proportionate to its degree of denfity; and this denfity decreafes in a certain ratio, according to its diftance from the furface of the earth. Rain therefore in its defcent will be every inftant acquiring an acceffion to the bulk of its drops, by attracting thefe aqueous vapours. For the cold produced by a falling fhower, will precipitate from the air, both its diffolved and diffufed water. And thus, at different heights, will be produced, from this caufe, fome difference in the quantity of rain which falls over the fame fpot of ground. The difcharge of the electrical fluid from a falling fhower, may alfo act as a powerful precipitant of the vapours, which are chemically diffolved in the

(c) It has been obferved to be fair, on the top of the cathedral at York, when there were fmall drizzling rains, with thick mifts, in the ftreets below. See Georgical Effays, p. 112.

the air. For by conveying an electrified wire to the surface of a quantity of water, saturated with any saline substance, an immediate and copious precipitation is produced, and the salt forms itself into large *flocculi*.

RAIN, when undisturbed by winds, descends in lines converging towards the centre of the earth, like the *radii* of a circle. This direction towards the perpendicular, however trifling in degree, gives some little tendency to the drops to coalesce together, and concurs in the general effect of producing a different quantity of rain at different heights.

FROM what has been advanced, it appears probable to me, that the gradual discharge of the electrical fire is the principal cause of the phænomenon I have attempted to explain. As the rain descends, the drops coalesce more and more together, by the continued diminution of the repulsive power which counteracted their mutual attraction; and consequently, in a given space, a much larger quantity will fall near to, than at a distance from the surface of the earth. A cloud which fills many thousand acres in the higher regions of the air, when the electric fluid operates upon it with full force, may not cover one third of that extent, when it has descended in a shower of rain. To this effect, the precipitation of the vapours contained in a dissolved

or

or diffused state, in the lower regions of the atmosphere, and the influence of gravitation, in producing a convergency of the drops of rain, will, in some degree, contribute.

POSTSCRIPT.

HAVING communicated the preceding paper to several of my literary friends, I have been favoured by Dr. Watson with the following curious fact.——"The water in the rain-"gauge at the top of Lord Charles Cavendish's "and Doctor Heberden's houses, which are "about a mile distant from each other, pretty "nearly correspond; but at the bottom of Lord "Charles's house, though the level is forty feet "above the top of Doctor Heberden's, the "quantity always exceeds that of Doctor Heber-"den's. Last year, for instance, at the top of "both their houses, there were collected about "twenty-two inches of rain; but in Lord "Charles's garden, at a distance from any "buildings, there fell twenty-six inches; and "this in his Lordship's garden has been constant "for several years. Doctor Heberden has been "too much confined to make accurate observa-"tions at the bottom of his late house; but he is "now

"now removed to Pall Mall, where his oppor-"tunities of obſerving are more favourable."

This fact, at firſt ſight, appears to be a ſtrong objection to the *hypotheſis* I have advanced. May it not, however, be obviated by ſuppoſing, that the diſcharge of the electrical fluid from a falling ſhower, is not ſo much influenced by the abſolute, as by the relative height of the places where the rain deſcends? And as the earth may be conſidered as the great recipient and attractor of electrical fire; is it not probable, that the quantity of rain collected, will be proportionate to the diſtance of the receiver from the ground immediately below, and not to its abſolute height, meaſured from any diſtant level, except in ſuch altitudes, where the denſity of the air, and the vapours floating in it, are ſo far diminiſhed as to produce a ſenſible variation? But I offer this conjecture with diffidence; and am ſenſible indeed, that the whole of my attempt to account for the different quantities of rain, which fall at different heights, is liable to objections, becauſe the *data* are yet few upon which it is founded. To promote the ſolution of ſo curious a *phænomenon*, I ſhall here ſubjoin a few queries, propoſed to me by different correſpondents. The fourth ſhould, I apprehend, be reverſed; becauſe it appears probable to me, that trees, plants, water, and moiſt earth, afford more copious

copious exhalations than paved ſtreets, houſes, burning fuel, or the bodies of men.

I. Does a glaſs funnel catch an equal quantity of rain, at the ſame height, as a metal funnel; the former being an electric, the latter a non-electric?

II. Is there a difference in the quantity of rain and ſnow catched in ſimilar veſſels, at different heights?

III. Is the difference of rain, catched at different heights, greateſt at the beginning of a ſhower?

IV. Is not this difference greater in large cities, than in the country, owing to the lower regions of the air being more loaded with watery vapours, which have been exhaled by fires, and from the human body?

V. Has the wind no ſhare in producing the diſparity obſerved in the quantities of rain, which fall at different heights?

VI. May not the column of air through which a drop of rain paſſes, in the ſpace of twenty or thirty yards, contain a ſufficient quantity of watery particles, to double the bulk of the drop? This may be illuſtrated by precipitating any ſaline ſubſtance from a ſaturated ſolution of it, contained in a cylindrical veſſel, and examining the proportional quantities of precipitate at different heights. Or, perhaps, it may be

 determined

determined by the following experiment: Take a cylindrical glaſs veſſel, four inches in diameter, and eight inches high; fill it with ice or ſnow, and place it in a warm room. A watery dew will ſoon be congealed upon its ſurface, which, being committed to a nice ſcale, may probably be found to be equal in gravity to a drop of rain. Suppoſe this cylinder to be drawn out to the length of twenty or thirty yards; the ſurface of it will ſtill continue nearly the ſame, though the diameter be diminiſhed; and ſuch a tube will aptly repreſent the column of air, through which a drop of rain deſcends, in its paſſage to the earth.

MARCH 30, 1771.

EXTRACT *of a* LETTER *from* BENJAMIN FRANKLIN, LL.D. &c. *(a)*

"ON my return to London I found your favour, of the ſixteenth of May (1771). I wiſh I could, as you deſire, give you a better explana-

(a) I truſt my friend Dr. Franklin will forgive the liberty I take, in communicating the following letter, with which I was honoured by him, on this occaſion. The opinions and conjectures of ſo eminent a philoſopher may, almoſt, be deemed common property; and on the point in queſtion, they are of peculiar value and authority.

tion

tion of the phænomenon in queſtion, ſince you ſeem not quite ſatisfied with your own; but I think we want more and a greater variety of experiments, in different circumſtances, to enable us to form a thoroughly ſatisfactory hypotheſis. Not that I make the leaſt doubt of the facts already related, as I know both Lord Charles Cavendiſh, and Dr. Heberden to be very accurate experimenters: But I wiſh to know the event of the trials propoſed in your ſix queries; and alſo, whether, in the ſame place where the lower veſſel receives nearly twice the quantity of water that is received by the upper, a third veſſel, placed at half the height, will receive a quantity proportionable. I will, however, endeavour to explain to you what occurred to me, when I firſt heard of the fact.

I SUPPOSE, it will be generally allowed, on a little conſideration of the ſubject, that ſcarce any drop of water was, when it began to fall from the clouds, of a magnitude equal to that it has acquired, when it arrives at the earth; the ſame of the ſeveral pieces of hail; becauſe they are often ſo large and weighty, that we cannot conceive a poſſibility of their being ſuſpended in the air, and remaining at reſt there, for any time, how ſmall ſoever; nor do we conceive any means of forming them ſo large, before they ſet out to fall. It ſeems then, that each beginning drop,

 and

and particle of hail receives continual addition in its progreſs downwards: This may be ſeveral ways: By the union of numbers in their courſe, ſo that what was at firſt only a deſcending miſt, becomes a ſhower; or, by each particle, in its deſcent through air that contains a great quantity of diſſolved water, ſtriking againſt, attaching to itſelf, and carrying down with it ſuch particles of that diſſolved water, as happen to be in its way; or attracting to itſelf ſuch as do not lie directly in its courſe, by its different ſtate with regard either to common or electric fire; or by all theſe cauſes united.

In the firſt caſe, by the uniting of numbers, larger drops might be made, but the quantity falling in the ſame ſpace would be the ſame, at all heights; unleſs, as you mention, the whole ſhould be contracted in falling, the lines deſcribed by all the drops converging, ſo that what ſet out to fall from a cloud of many thouſand acres, ſhould reach the earth in perhaps a third of that extent; of which I ſomewhat doubt. In the other caſes we have two experiments.

1. A dry glaſs bottle, filled with very cold water, in a warm day, will preſently collect, from the ſeemingly dry air that ſurrounds it, a quantity of water that ſhall cover its ſurface and run down its ſides, which perhaps is done by the power wherewith the cold water attracts the

the fluid, common fire, that had been united with the diſſolved water in the air, and drawing that fire through the glaſs into itſelf, leaves the water on the outſide.

2. An electrified body left in a room, for ſome time, will be more covered with duſt than other bodies, in the ſame room, not electrified, which duſt ſeems to be attracted from the circumambient air.

Now we know, that the rain, even in our hotteſt days, comes from a very cold region. Its falling ſometimes in the form of ice, ſhews this clearly; and perhaps even the rain is ſnow or ice when it firſt moves downwards, though thawed in falling: And we know that the drops of rain are often electrified: But thoſe cauſes of addition to each drop of water, or piece of hail, one would think, could not long continue to produce the ſame effect; ſince the air, through which the drops fall, muſt ſoon be ſtript of its previouſly diſſolved water, ſo as to be no longer capable of augmenting them. Indeed very heavy ſhowers, of either, are never of long continuance; but moderate rains often continue ſo long as to puzzle this hypotheſis: So that, upon the whole, I think, as I intimated before, that we are yet hardly ripe for making one."

ESSAY IV.

ON THE SOLUTION OF HUMAN CALCULI BY FIXED AIR.

I FLATTER myſelf, that fixed air is now become an object of the attention of phyſicians; as it has been fully ſhewn that it is capble of being applied to many important medicinal purpoſes. In *pulmonic diſorders*, the *gangrenous ſore throat*, and in *malignant fevers*, the happieſt effects have been experienced from the uſe of it; and I know not a more powerful remedy for *foul ulcers*, as it mitigates pain, promotes a good digeſtion, and corrects the putrid diſpoſition of the fluids. I have related ſeveral caſes, in the former volume, and in the Appendix to Dr. Prieſtley's Treatiſe on Air, which evince the truth of theſe obſervations; and ſince their

their firſt publication, a variety of ſimilar facts have occurred to my learned friend Dr. Dobſon, in his hoſpital practice at Leverpool; and to Dr. Rotherham, at Newcaſtle upon Tyne.

But I have a farther, and very intereſting diſcovery to communicate, concerning the medicinal properties of this ſpecies of factitious air. About the end of laſt year, I was informed, that doctor Saunders, a phyſician in London, eminent for his knowledge of chemiſtry, had employed it as a ſolvent of the human *calculus.* I was ignorant of the manner in which his trials were conducted, and of the ſucceſs which had attended them; but my curioſity was excited; the acquiſition of ſuch a remedy was flattering to my hopes; and I engaged in the purſuit of it almoſt with as much ardour, as if it had been the philoſopher's ſtone. I recollected, that Dr. Black and Mr. Cavendiſh have proved the ſolubility of various earthy bodies in water, either by abſtracting from, or ſuperadding to the fixed air which they contain: And as the human *calculus* is diſſolved in the former way, by lime water, and the cauſtic alkali; it appeared highly probable, that the like effect would be produced, on the ſame ſubſtance, by the latter mode of operation. Analogy ſeemed favourable to the hypotheſis, and experiment has confirmed it.

Experiment I. December 13, 1774. A human *calculus*, in figure and ſize like a Piſtachio nut, of a ſmooth ſurface and firm texture, and which weighed fifty-two grains, was ſuſpended in pure ſpring water, ſtrongly impregnated with fixed air, and continually ſupplied with freſh ſtreams of it, by an elegant and well contrived apparatus, lately invented *(a)*. After forty-eight hours maceration, the ſtone was carefully dried, and weighed forty-nine grains and a half. It was become more friable in its texture.

Experiment II. Another *calculus*, extracted from the ſame bladder, and ſimilar to the former in figure, texture, and in the ſmoothneſs of its ſurface, was immerſed, forty-eight hours, in a quantity of the ſpring water before employed, not impregnated with fixed air. The weight of the ſtone, before immerſion, was forty-two grains and a half; and after it was taken out of the water, and thoroughly dried, forty-two grains. The texture and external appearance of it were unchanged.

Experiment III. The *calculus* employed in the firſt experiment, and which now weighed forty-nine grains and a half, was ſuſpended, during the ſpace of forty-eight hours, in an

(a) By Dr. Nooth, and ſold by Parker, glaſs-man, Fleet-Street, London.

atmoſphere

atmoſphere of fixed air, and expoſed to a ſtream of it, at the diſtance of ſeven inches from the effervefcing mixture of chalk, water, and oil of vitriol. By this operation the *calculus* was rendered much more friable; the *laminæ* of which it was compoſed were looſened, and part of the external one was ſeparated; its colour was changed from grey to white, and, when committed to the balance, it weighed fifty-one grains, having abſorbed a grain and a half of fixed air. By expoſure, during the night, to the common atmoſphere, the ſtone loſt half a grain of this additional weight, and another half grain afterwards by being laid before the fire.

EXPERIMENT IV. Three *calculi* were ſuſpended in an atmoſphere of fixed air, and expoſed, as in the laſt experiment, to a ſtream of it, during three days. When put into the veſſel, the firſt was of a yellow colour, and ſolid texture, and weighed two drachms, forty-five grains and a half. By the abſorption of fixed air, its gravity was increaſed above the third part of a grain; the colour, in certain ſpots, was rendered lighter, and thoſe ſpots were ſofter than other parts of the ſtone. The ſecond *calculus* was of a white colour, and cryſtallized form; and weighed, before immerſion in the fixed air, two drachms, ſix grains and a half. Its weight, when taken out of the veſſel, was unchanged; but

but the ſurface of it was become more friable than before. The third ſtone was one drachm, eight grains and a half; was hard, and of a bright colour; and the external *laminæ* of it were broken. It acquired half a grain from the fixed air, and was rendered ſomewhat ſofter and whiter.

EXPERIMENT V. The *calculi* employed in the foregoing experiment were immerſed, three days, in mephitic water, conſtantly ſupplied with freſh ſtreams of fixed air, by the apparatus before mentioned. Each ſtone was then thoroughly dried, and expoſed, forty-eight hours, in damp weather, to the air of my ſtudy, before the weight of it was examined. Number one, the yellow *calculus*, was changed to a very light colour, almoſt approaching to white, and had loſt more than two grains. Number two was become perfectly white in many parts, was very friable, and had loſt one grain and a half. Number three was rendered white in various parts; was more friable, and was diminiſhed in weight three grains and a half.

THESE experiments fully evince, that water impregnated with fixed air is a powerful diſſolvent of the human *calculus*. And it is probable, that the action of this *menſtruum* would have been conſiderably increaſed, if a proper degree of heat could have been employed. Even the

the warmth of ſummer might have proved favourable to my trials; which were made in a ſeaſon, when the greateſt height to which the mercury roſe in the thermometer, was the fifty-fourth degree of Fahrenheit's ſcale. Lime water has been long and juſtly celebrated as a lithontriptic; but its ſolvent powers appear to be inferior to the artificial mineral water, of which we are now treating. As a proof of this, it may not be improper to relate the following experiment, although it was made on a different occaſion, and is inſerted in the former volume *(b)*.

EXPERIMENT VI. Three fragments of human *calculi*, numbered for the ſake of diſtinction, one, two, three, were immerſed in equal quantities of different lime waters; the firſt in lime water made with diſtilled water, the ſecond in lime water prepared with hard pump water, and the third in lime water made with the ſame hard pump water, poured, boiling hot, upon the quick lime. Number one was of a brown colour, and hard texture; was ſmooth on one ſide, and rough on the other; and weighed twenty-ſix grains and a half. Number two was a fragment of the ſame *calculus*, and weighed twenty-five grains and a half. Number three,

(b) See vol. I. Eſſay VI. p. 173.

a fragment

a fragment of a different *calculus*, was of a loofer and more fpongy texture than the former, and weighed twenty-feven grains. The phials which contained the *calculi*, and four ounces, by meafure, of lime water, were all nearly full, and clofely corked. After continuing the maceration, eight days, without heat, the *calculi* were taken out, carefully dried, on filtering paper, before a gentle fire, and then weighed. Number one had loft a grain and a half, and was covered, in many parts, with a foft, white, cretaceous matter. Number two had loft only half a grain: Many little cryftals fhot from its furface. Number three had loft a grain: But it fhould be remarked, that this fragment was much fofter than the other two.

Experiment VII. Three drachms of the cauftic alkali, prepared by Mr. Lane, rendered a pint of water fo pungent, that the tongue and palate could fcarcely endure the tafte of it. In this liquor were macerated, forty-eight hours, two *calculi*, one of which weighed a hundred and forty-one grains, the other thirty-three grains and a quarter. When dried, the firft ftone had loft four grains and three quarters, the *laminæ* of it were feparated in many places, and it was covered with a white efflorefcence. The fecond ftone fuffered a diminution in weight of three grains; one of its *laminæ* was feparated; and a white

white efflorefcence alfo appeared on the furface of it. The water, impregnated with the cauftic alkali, was defended from the atmofphere, during the experiment; but had acquired, from the *calculi*, fuch a quantity of fixed air, as to effervefce with the acid of vitriol.

EXPERIMENT VIII. A fimilar experiment was tried with two other *calculi*, which were immerfed, during the fame fpace of time, in a pint of water ftrongly acidulated with oil of vitriol. One of the *calculi*, which weighed a hundred and fixty-five grains, was unchanged in its appearance, and diminifhed in weight fcarcely half a grain. The other ftone was rendered very friable, had a white efflorefcence in feveral parts of it, and was reduced from forty-one to thirty-one grains.

HUMAN CALCULI vary in their ftructure and compofition; and it has been fhewn, by Dr. Dawfon *(c)*, that fome of them, which are foluble in an alkaline, are but little affected by an acid *menftruum*; whilft others will refift the action of an alkali, and yet be readily diffolved by an acid. Even in the fame fubject, he obferves, there may be found *calculi* of oppofite kinds, fome of which will diffolve in acids, fome in alkalis, and fome in neither; as, from careful and fufficient

(c) See the Medical Tranfactions, vol. II. p. 105.

trials

trials, he judged to be the caſe in a patient of his own. But water impregnated with fixed air, though inferior in efficacy to the vitriolic acid, or the cauſtic alkali, is a more univerſal ſolvent than either of them. For, as far as my obſervations have reached, it acts upon every *calculus* that is ſuſpended in it. And I have tried it with thoſe which have ſuffered no diminution of weight from the *menſtrua* above-mentioned. But a farther detail of my experiments would be no leſs tedious than unneceſſary. And I flatter myſelf, that I may now, without incurring the imputation of enthuſiaſm, expreſs the heart-felt ſatisfaction I enjoy, in the diſcovery of a new lithontriptic medicine, that is at once grateful to the palate, ſtrengthening to the ſtomach, and ſalutary to the whole ſyſtem. Lime water often nauſeates the patient, deſtroys his appetite, and creates the heart-burn; and the ſoap ley is ſo cauſtic and acrimonious, that it can be taken only in the ſmalleſt quantity, frequently produces bloody urine, and aggravates the tortures it is intended to relieve. Both theſe remedies alſo require a very ſtrict regimen of diet; and their qualities are liable to be changed either by acidities, or the fermentation of our food in the firſt paſſages. But the mephitic water may be drunk in the largeſt quantity, without ſatiety or inconvenience: It requires no reſtrictions in diet, and

and its medicinal virtues will be undiminiſhed in the ſtomach or bowels.

Perhaps it may be queſtioned, whether fixed air can be conveyed, by the ordinary courſe of circulation, to the kidneys and bladder. In an elaſtic ſtate, it certainly cannot; but diſſolved in water, it may paſs through the vaſcular ſyſtem without creating the leaſt diſturbance or diſorder, and, by its diuretic quality, will be powerfully determined to the urinary organs. So ſtrong is the relation that ſubſiſts between mephitic air and water, that they remain firmly combined, although expoſed to conſiderable variations of heat and cold. Dr. Prieſtley found, that it required half an hour, even when the boiling heat was employed, to expel completely the fixed air from a phial of impregnated water; and I have obſerved, that it has retained its peculiar flavour ſeveral days, when left in a baſon, with a large ſurface open to the external air.

Experiment IX. But to obtain more ſatiſfactory evidence upon this ſubject, I filled a bottle with mephitic air, and placed it in a heat of about ninety-eight degrees of Fahrenheit's thermometer. A bent glaſs tube, a quarter of an inch in diameter, properly luted at each end, formed a communication between this bottle and one of lime water; to the bottom of which it extended. An inteſtine motion ſoon enſued;

air

air bubbles were ſlowly conveyed into the lime water; and a white precipitation was gradually formed. In an hour and a half, the lime water was become turbid, but was quickly rendered quite milky by blowing air into it from the lungs. The mephitic water ſtill retained its volatile and acidulous taſte; and when a greater degree of heat (108°) was applied to the bottle which contained it, a briſk inteſtine motion was renewed.

EXPERIMENT X. A ſmall quantity of mephitic air, which had been expoſed ten days to the atmoſphere, in a phial uncorked, ſtill retained its acidulous taſte; and when immerſed in water heated to a hundred and forty degrees of Fahrenheit's thermometer, emitted air bubbles very copiouſly. The phial remained in the water till it ceaſed to diſcharge any air; but a very ſlight agitation again renewed the inteſtine motion; and it rendered lime water, when mixed with it, as white as milk.

THE judicious writer, to whoſe uſeful paper I have before referred, has recommended an attention to the fragments, ſcales, or films, which the ſtone in the kidneys or bladder may caſt off, and alſo to the contents and ſediment of the urine; that a diſcovery may be made, whether the proper ſolvent be an acid, or an alkaline *menſtruum*. If it appear to be the former,

mer, the elixir of vitriol may be uſed in conjunction with mephitic water, to which it will be no ungrateful or inſalutary addition. And there is reaſon to believe, that this acid may be conveyed to the kidneys, without any conſiderable change in its properties. It is not ſubject to fermentation, and is diſpoſed to paſs off by urine. The ſucceſsful exhibition of it in the itch, ſeems to evince, that it is capable of being received into the vaſcular ſyſtem, and of being excreted, probably in a volatilized ſtate, by the pores of the ſkin. Even when given to nurſes, labouring under this complaint, it is ſaid both to cure them, and the children whom they ſuckle *(d)*.

As the vapour of chalk and oil of vitriol has been found ſo efficacious in correcting the *ſanies*, and abating the pain of foul ulcers, when externally applied; we may reaſonably preſume, that the internal uſe of the ſame remedy will prove beneficial, in ſimilar affections of the urinary paſſages. Such complaints frequently occur in practice, and may ariſe, either from *calculi* in the kidneys and bladder; from the receſſion of ſcor

(d) Vide Diſſertationem de Olei Vitrioli uſu in quibuſdam Scabiei ſpeciebus. 1762. Medical and Philoſophical Commentaries, vol. I. p. 103

butic eruptions; from the venereal diſeaſe; from ſtrains; centuſions; or various other cauſes. And water impregnated with fixed air ſeems well adapted, by its diuretic, healing, and antiſeptic powers, to waſh off and ſweeten the acrid matter; to abate the defluxion on the mucous membrane; to contract the flabby edges of the ulcers; and to diſpoſe them to a ſpeedy granulation. If the pain, inflammation, and abſorption of the *pus* have excited a hectic fever, the patient may drink plentifully of Seltzer water, which is of a cooling quality, although it abounds with mephitic air; or a ſmall quantity of Rochelle ſalt may be added to the mineral water artificially prepared. Thus will the increaſed action of the heart and arteries, which may ariſe from the ſtimulus of the fixed air, be entirely obviated, without the leaſt diminution of its medicinal powers. And whilſt the ſanction of experience is wanting, reaſon will juſtify the trial of a remedy, which is at once ſafe, pleaſant, and efficacious.

In ulcers of the kidneys and bladder, the urine is commonly high coloured, pungent, and of an offenſive ſmell. To aſcertain whether fixed air would correct theſe qualities, I attempted the following diſagreeable experiment.

Experiment XI. Repeated ſtreams of fixed air were conveyed into three pints of urine, which

which had been kept till it was become very putrid, and which emitted a ſtrong, volatile odour. I examined the ſmell of it, from time to time, whilſt this proceſs was carrying on, and compared it with a portion of the ſame urine, which was reſerved as a ſtandard. The pungency of it gradually abated; it acquired a brighter colour and was leſs turbid, but its putrid odour ſeemed to be increaſed. Theſe obſervations were made in the evening, and, early the next morning, I awoke with a violent head-ach, which was attended with vomiting and a diarrhœa. Alarmed at theſe effects, which I attributed to the putrid vapours of the urine, I dropt the proſecution of the experiment; but the ſucceeding day, Mr. Thomas Smith, a young gentleman who will one day be an ornament to the profeſſion of phyſic, undertook the examination which I had begun: And, after attentively comparing the ſtandard and the urine impregnated with fixed air, he found the latter more offenſively putrid than the former, but without any degree of pungency, or volatility. As this experiment was not completed, I am uncertain whether the urine was ſweetened by the mephitic air. But it is evident, that the volatile alkali, generated by putrefaction, was either neutralized, diſſipated, or prevented from aſcending, by the atmoſphere of fixed air, which filled the other part of the veſſel. Perhaps this atmoſphere might be the *menſtruum* of the putrid *effluvia* emitted by the urine, which being then accumulated, would appear to have its *fœtor* increaſed. In another work, I have related an experiment, made by my friend Mr. Henry, ſomewhat ſimilar to this, and which ſuggeſted to him the like explanation. A piece of putrid fleſh was ſuſpended, twelve hours, in a three pint bottle, cloſely corked, and filled with fixed air, which had been ſeparated from chalk by the vitriolic acid. The beef was conſiderably ſweetened, but the air in the bottle was rendered intolerably offenſive.

THE waters of Bath, in Somerſetſhire, have been long and juſtly celebrated for their efficacy in the jaundice and other hepatic diſorders. They abound with fixed air; and it may be of importance, to aſcertain whether they derive from this active principle, the power of diſſolving the concretions of the bile, and of removing the obſtructions in the liver. I was induced, therefore, to try the ſolubility of gall ſtones in mephitic water. But I have as yet, only a ſolitary experiment on the ſubject, to offer to the reader.

EXPERIMENT XII. A gall ſtone, that had been extracted from a tumour in the region of the liver, was divided into two parts. One of theſe

these, which weighed fifty-one grains and a half, was immersed, four days, in rain water strongly impregnated with fixed air. The other weighed twenty grains and a quarter, and was macerated in simple rain water, during the same space of time. The first fragment, when carefully dried, was become heavier by one grain, having gained so much from the fixed air. In texture and appearance, it remained unchanged. The second fragment had lost one eighth of a grain.

I MEAN not to draw any decisive inference from a single experiment: But it is probable, that the Bath waters resolve concretions of the bile, not so much by a chemical operation, as by accelerating the secretions of the liver, stimulating the organs of digestion, and invigorating the whole animal system. Nature, indeed, observes a peculiar œconomy in the circulation of the blood through the liver; and, as the bile is one of her most elaborate fluids, it must be difficult to introduce a foreign and unassimilated substance into it. From analogy, however, we may conclude, that this is not impracticable. The milk and the saliva are frequently impregnated with adventitious matters; and these animal liquors, like the bile, are secreted by organs of a particular structure, and for determinate and important purposes. A remedy which would pass unchanged into the system of the liver, and medicate the bile ſo as to render it unapt to coagulate, or enable it to reſolve the concretions already formed, would be a moſt valuable acquiſition(e). And the obſtacles to the attainment of it ſhould rather be regarded as incitements to our induſtry, than apologies for ſupineneſs and deſpair. Such, it muſt be acknowledged, they have proved; as appears from the variety of diſſolvents which have been propoſed, and tried. Acids, alkalis, ſoap, ardent and dulcified ſpirits, with freſh vegetable juices, have been recommended. Valiſnerius found, that a compoſition of alcohol and oil of turpentine deſtroyed the texture and coheſion of gall ſtones, more perfectly than any other *menſtruum*(f); and Mr. William White, of York, has fully confirmed this obſervation, by a number of judicious experiments which he has communicated to me. Some time ago, I thought favourably of this remedy, and endeavoured to promote the trial of it(g); but farther reflection has convinced me, that the continued uſe of it is more likely to prove injurious than beneficial. Spirituous liquors, of all ſorts, have a peculiarly unfavourable operation on the liver; and it would be abſurd to ſeek a *ſpecific medicine* for the diſeaſes of

(e) Vide Medical Tranſactions, vol. II. p. 165.

(f) Tom. III. p. 6. (g) See vol. I. p. 427.

of the bile, in what experience has fatally ſhewn to be a *ſpecific poiſon* to the organ which ſecretes it. Perhaps fixed air, under ſome form or other, may hereafter be found to be the *deſideratum* which we have been ſo long purſuing. At leaſt, we may be allowed to attribute ſome ſhare of the virtues which the Bath waters poſſeſs, to this ingredient in their compoſition; and when they cannot be employed, to recommend the mephitic water, as an innocent and efficacious ſubſtitute.

FROM the obſervations advanced in the preceding eſſay, it appears highly *probable*, that fixed air may be conveyed, by the ordinary courſe of circulation, to the kidneys and bladder. But I can now ſpeak *deciſively* concerning this intereſting point. For the young gentleman before-mentioned has, at my deſire, taken large quantities of mephitic water daily, during the ſpace of a fortnight. And whilſt he continued this courſe, his urine was ſtrongly impregnated with fixed air,. as appeared from the precipitation which it produced in lime water; from the bubbles which it copiouſly emitted when placed under the receiver of an air pump; and from the ſolution of ſeveral urinary ſtones, which were immerſed in it.

DR. PRIESTLEY's favourable opinion of this new lithontriptic medicine may be collected from the following paragraphs, which I have extracted from the ſecond volume of his Experiments and Obſervations on air, p. 216.

"IT might be queſtioned, whether the fixed air "contained in our aliments can be conveyed, by "the courſe of circulation, into the blood, and, "by that means, impregnate the urine. I have "found, however, that it may do it; having "more than once expelled, from a quantity of "freſh made urine, by means of heat, about "one fifth of its bulk of pure fixed air, as ap-"peared by its precipitating lime in lime water, "and being almoſt wholly abſorbed by water; "and yet a very good air pump did not diſcover "that it contained any air at all.

"IT muſt be obſerved, however, that it re-"quired ſeveral hours to expel this air by heat; "and, after the proceſs, there was a conſider-"able whitiſh ſediment at the bottom of the "veſſel. This was probably ſome calcareous "matter, with which the fixed air had been "united; and, by this fixed air, the calcareous "matter, which would otherwiſe have formed "a ſtone or gravel, may have been held in ſo-"lution. And, therefore, drinking water im-"pregnated

" pregnated with fixed air, may, by impreg-" nating the urine, enable it to diſſolve calcare-" ous matters better than it would otherwiſe have" done; and may, therefore, be a means of pre-" venting or diſſolving the ſtone in the bladder," agreeably to the propoſal of my friend Dr." Percival."

Sir John Pringle informs me, that he has known great benefit to accrue from the uſe of honey, in caſes of the gravel, or when the kidneys are loaded with ſand. He directs about a pound and a quarter of this remedy to be taken every week, and continued for a conſiderable ſpace of time. And, as it perfectly coincides with the artificial mineral water, being diuretic and containing much fixed air, he recommends to me the trial of them together. My readers will, I doubt not, be much pleaſed with this valuable hint *(b)*.

These

(b) Sir John Pringle, in a ſubſequent letter, dated December 28, 1776, ſays, " I recommend a continuation of the honey, for life, both in the gravel and in " the periodic aſthma (ſuch as Floyer deſcribes his caſe to " have been); and that the quantity be from a pound to " a pound and a quarter in the week; that is, to thoſe of " a puny make, and to women, I direct the pound, and " to the more robuſt, twenty ounces. Mr. Hume, one of " the commiſſioners of the ſick and wounded, has conſumed, regularly, for theſe fourteen years paſt, five pounds " of

THESE obſervations, on the medicinal and lithontriptic qualities of fixed air, may now be regarded as practical truths, which have been eſtabliſhed by experience. Since the publication of the foregoing experiments (*i*), I have had the moſt incontrovertible evidence, that this remedy alleviates the ſymptoms both of the ſtone and gravel; that it acts as a powerful diuretic; diſcharges ſabulous concretions; heals ulcerations in the urinary paſſages; invigorates the organs of digeſtion; and ſtrengthens the whole ſyſtem. In ſaying ſo much, I am warranted by my own experience, which has been confirmed by ſimilar obſervations, tranſmitted to me from various parts

" (of ſixteen ounces each), every month; and ſince the " third or fourth month from the commencement of this " courſe, he has not had one return of that kind of aſthma, " with which he had been ſo much troubled before, even for " the ſpace of ſixteen years. The honey was begun for this " diſtemper; but, as he happened to be likewiſe liable to " very painful paroxyſms of the gravel, he was agreeably " ſurprized to find, that he received almoſt as much benefit " from his medicine, in this ailment as in the other. From " having had a nephritic attack, and paſſing ſand and ſmall " ſtones, for ſome years, once in one, two, or three months, " before taking the honey, he has had, in the laſt fourteen " years, but two or three in all; and, although he has, " in one or two of them, voided a ſmall calculus, yet it was " with ſcarcely any pain."

(*i*) See a Letter to the Editor of the Medical Commentaries, vol. V. p. 176, alſo p. 448, for the year 1777.

parts of England. But it is difficult to *afcertain* the folution of a ftone in the bladder, by any medicine; and it cannot, therefore, be deemed extraordinary, that I have yet feen no decifive cafe, in the circle of my practice, of the complete efficacy of this new folvent. A phyfician of eminence, in London, has, however, been more fuccefsful; having brought away, to ufe his own words in a letter to me, in fmall fragments, and in a whitifh chalk-like fubftance, a ftone from the urinary bladder, by adminiftering fixed air to his patient, during the fpace of a few weeks. The hiftory of this cafe has been offered to the public by Dr. Hulme, with feveral others, which, though lefs certain and important, tend to evince the lithontriptic action of fixed air. And another refpectable phyfician, Dr. Saunders, has lately given the following teftimony of the fame remedy. "I am fully con- "vinced, from a variety of trials, that water "impregnated with the mephitic acid is carried "unchanged to the human bladder; and, that "this remedy has done great fervice in calculous "complaints." But, when fixed air is employed as a diffolvent of the ftone, the ufe of it muft generally be continued for many months. Relief is often obtained by it in a fhorter time; but few cafes will occur, like the one recorded by Dr. Hulme, in which the calculus appears to have been of a remarkably ſoft and friable texture. The reputation of the moſt efficacious remedies is frequently injured by the unwarrantable expectations of mankind concerning them. And, in chronic diſorders, many a cure is deſpaired of, which might be accompliſhed by more patience in the ſick, and greater perſeverance in the practitioner.

DIRECTIONS *for* ADMINISTERING FIXED AIR *in* CASES *of the* STONE *or* GRAVEL.

GIVE the patient, every ſixth hour, three ounces of the *aqua mephitica alkalina*, prepared according to the directions of Mr. Bewly *(k)*, and ſweeten it, to the taſte, with honey. Direct him to drink, at proper intervals, a glaſs of the mephitic water, acidulated with the *ſpiritus vitrioli tenuis*, and ſweetened with honey. Two or three pints of this beverage ſhould be conſumed in twenty-four hours; and, indeed, it is ſo pleaſant, that it may be taken at meals, with or without the addition of a little wine. In lieu of the mephitic alkaline water, half a drachm of ſalt of tartar may be diſſolved in three ounces of ſimple water, ſweetened, to the palate, with honey, to which half an ounce of freſh lemon juice muſt be added, at the

(k) Prieſtley on Air, vol. II. p. 346.

time

time when the draught is ſwallowed. The lemon juice will neutralize about one ſcruple of the alkali, expelling the fixed air which it contained; and this fixed air will combine partly with the water, and partly with the remaining ten grains of unneutralized alkali.

IF honey agree with the bowels of the patient, it may be taken at pleaſure. Cyder, perry, briſk fermenting wines, and bottled beer, all contain much fixed air, and may, therefore, be temperately uſed, as they coincide with the courſe here directed. If the patient be coſtive, magneſia alba uncalcined will be the beſt purgative. If he be too lax, the chalk julep of the London Diſpenſatory may be preſcribed *(l)*.

(l) Theſe directions were inſerted in the Medical Commentaries for the year 1777. In 1784, if I miſtake not, the ACCOUNT *of the efficacy of the* AQUA MEPHITICA ALKALINA, *in calculous diſorders,* was publiſhed by Dr. Falconer, from the M.SS. of Dr. Dobſon.

ESSAY

ESSAY V.

EXPERIMENTS AND OBSERVATIONS ON THE NATURE AND COMPOSITION OF URINARY CALCULI.

A CALCULUS, extracted from a young man about two years ago, by my friend Mr. Charles White, of Manchester, had so much the appearance of chalk, that I was induced to make some experiments upon it. The *nucleus* was a bougie, which had unfortunately passed into the bladder; and a stone, of considerable size, had been formed in less than twelve months.

EXPERIMENT I. A few grains of this *calculus* produced a strong effervescence with thirty drops of oil of vitriol, and half an ounce of water. Thirty-eight grains of it were calcined in a crucible, placed, two hours, in a wind furnace; and to this *calx*, which weighed twenty-four grains, were

were added five ounces of water. The water acquired a ſlight impregnation of quick lime; and, after filtration, depoſited a ſmall ſediment, when a ſtream of fixed air was conveyed into it.

Experiment II. In the laſt experiment, the portion of the *calculus* employed was probably too ſmall, to give more than a ſlight impregnation to ſo many ounces of water. Another ſtone, therefore, of a white colour, but which did not effervesce with oil of vitriol, was calcined in the ſame furnace, during the ſpace of *three hours*. By this proceſs, the *calculus* was reduced in weight from three hundred and nine, to ninety-two grains; and, though the ſolid particles ſcarcely impreſſed the tongue with any ſenſe of cauſticity, yet they communicated, to five ounces of water, a very ſtrong taſte of quick lime; and the filtered liquor became milky by blowing air into it from the lungs, and ſoon depoſited a large white ſediment.

Experiment III. A third *calculus*, of a cloſe texture and red colour, which did not effervesce with ſpirit of vitriol, and weighed ſeven drachms and a half, was put into the crucible, and, in a few hours, was entirely conſumed by the fire.

Experiment IV. A fourth *calculus*, in figure like a mulberry, and which did not effervesce with the vitriolic acid, was calcined three hours, and loſt more than three fifths of its weight by this

this proceſs. It taſted very acrid, and made a ſtrong lime water.

Experiment V. A fifth *calculus*, which weighed two hundred and forty-five grains before calcination, was reduced to thirty grains by this operation; and the remaining powder was taſteleſs, and gave no impregnation to water.

From theſe experiments we may conclude, that an abſorbent earth often enters into the compoſition of the urinary *calculus*. For it is the peculiar property of this claſs of bodies to be convertible into quick lime, by the action of fire. It does not ſeem probable, that this ſubſtance is the product of animalization, in the human ſpecies. The ſhells of ſea-fiſhes and of ſnails furniſh it, indeed, in large quantity; but the bones, horns, blood, ſkin and fleſh of animals, however ſtrongly calcined, are not changeable into lime. Mr. Rouelle has lately diſcovered the fixed alkali in the ſerum of the blood; and Dr. Lewis has obſerved, that the aſhes of fleſh and blood are readily, perfectly, and plentifully ſoluble in the mineral acids; and that they form with them an auſtere, aſtringent liquor, approaching to an aluminous nature *(a)*. The human *calculus* muſt, therefore, be conſidered as an heterogeneous ſubſtance, conſiſting of thoſe

(a) Lewis's Tranſlation of Newmann's Chemiſtry, p. 494.

recrementitious

recrementitious parts which are ſeparated from the blood, by the kidneys. Whether theſe parts differ eſſentially in different conſtitutions, or whether they vary, only, in the proportion which they bear to each other, is a point of difficult ſolution. I am inclined to adopt the latter ſuppoſition; but, however this may be decided, I think it is very evident, that *calculi* of the kidneys and bladder are not of animal original alone, as they frequently contain an abſorbent earth, which is not generated in the human body. This ſubſtance muſt, therefore, be conſidered as adventitious, and is probably conveyed into the ſyſtem by the uſe of HARD SPRING WATER, in which it commonly abounds. In a former work, I pointed out the pernicious effects of ſuch waters, in habits which are ſubject to the ſtone and gravel. But, influenced by the moſt reſpectable authorities *(b)*, I then believed, that the *calculi* of the urinary organs, partake not in the leaſt of a foſſil nature; and that their formation depends either upon ſome accidental *nucleus*; or upon a peculiar and often hereditary diſpoſition to concrete in the animal fluids. Hence I ſuppoſed, that impure waters were only *negatively* favourable to this diſpoſition, by having

(b) HIST. de l'Acad. Royale des Sciences, 1700. Perrault Vitruve, lib. VIII. c. 5. Medical Tranſactions, vol. I. p. 7. Sharp's Surgery, p. 75.

no tendency to diminish it. For water, whether used as nature presents us with it, or mixed with wine, or taken under the form of beer or ale, is the great diluter, vehicle, or solvent, both of our food, and of the saline, earthy, and superfluous parts of the animal juices. And it is more or less adapted to the performance of these offices, in proportion to its degree of purity; because a *menstruum* already loaded, and perhaps saturated with different contents, cannot act so powerfully, as one which is free from all sensible impregnation *(c)*. But, as an absorbent earth is found (Exp. I. II. IV.) to be often a component part of the human *calculus*, I am now convinced, that hard waters actually contribute to the formation of it. This is an opinion which the father of physic advanced, and which till lately has remained uncontroverted by his followers. *Damnantur imprimis fontes*, says Pliny, *quorum aquæ decoctæ, crassis obducunt vasa crustis (d)*. It was obvious indeed to infer, that waters which deposite a large earthy sediment, either in the aquæducts through which they are conveyed, or in the vessels in which they are boiled or preserved, would let fall their grosser particles in passing through the kidneys, and especially whilst retained in the bladder; and that these, by the continued

(c) See vol. I. p. 184. *(d)* Lib. XXXI. C. 3.

appposition

appoſition of freſh matter, connected by the animal *gluten*, and compacted by the action of thoſe organs, would form the ſtone or gravel. But the ſeparation of earthy matter in the urinary paſſages may be better explained by the chemical doctrine of affinities. For the vitriolic acid contained in *ſelenites*, with which hard ſpring waters are uſually impregnated, will forſake its baſis, and combine with the alkaline ſalts, ſo copiouſly diſcharged by thoſe excretories.

THAT the ſtone, though it is by no means a rare diſorder, does not more frequently occur in this country, which abounds with calcareous waters, is a difficulty which I muſt acknowledge myſelf at a loſs to obviate. But it may be remarked, that internal affections of the human body are ſeldom produced by a ſingle cauſe; and the concurrence of many may be neceſſary to form a *calculus* in the bladder *(e)*. This malady, however, is ſcarcely known in Switzerland, as I have lately been informed by a letter from Baron Haller. And the ſprings of that Alpine region are remarkably light, pure, and free from all mineral ingredients.

(e) Raro tamen ſimplex eſt, ſed plerumque ex pluribus conditionibus una concurrentibus compoſita. *Gaubii Pathologia. ſect.* 68.

In the ſecond and fourth experiments related above, the *calculi,* though they contained an abſorbent earth, did not effervеſce with the vitriolic acid. This muſt be aſcribed to the glutinous matter, in which the earthy particles were involved, and by which they were defended from the powerful action of the *menſtruum* employed.

April 1, 1775.

ESSAY VI.

EXPERIMENTS AND OBSERVATIONS ON THE EFFECTS OF FIXED AIR, ON THE COLOURS AND VEGETATION OF PLANTS (a).

THE influence of fixed air on vegetation is a new, curious, and very interefting object of inquiry. I was led into it, by a train of experiments, which the following paffage, in Dr. Prieftley's Obfervations on various kinds of Air, fuggefted to me. "A red rofe, frefh gathered, loft its rednefs, and became of a purple colour, after being held over fermenting liquor about twenty-four hours; but the tips of each leaf were much more affected than the reft of it. Another red rofe turned perfectly white in this fituation; but various other flowers, of

(a) Inferted in Dr. Hunter's Georgical Effays, p. 465.

different colours, were very little affected. These experiments were not repeated, as I wish they might be done, in pure fixed air, extracted from chalk by means of oil of vitriol."

March 16th, 1775. I EXPOSED a tulip, forty-eight hours, to a stream of fixed air, separated from chalk by means of oil of vitriol. The colours and odour were preserved unchanged; the leaves were curled at the edges, but remained firm and undecayed. Another tulip, gathered at the same time, from the same root, and similar in colour, soon became faded, flaccid, and lost its odour in the common atmosphere.

THE same experiment was made with a purple crocus; with a white and yellow jonquil; with the hepatica; with a polyanthus of a purple hue; and with a stock July flower. They were all perfectly preserved in the vessel of fixed air; whilst specimens of the same flowers speedily lost their bloom, and turned soft and shriveled in the open air.

THE Italian Narcissus, a delicate flower, which grew in a hot-house, retained its colours forty-eight hours in the fixed air; but the leaves of the flower cup were very much contracted.

A PALE red rose, taken from a hot-house, was exposed, twenty-four hours, to a stream of fixed air, without suffering any change of colour. It was

was carefully compared with another roſe, collected from the ſame tree *(a)*.

THE reſult of this experiment differs from that related by Dr. Prieſtley. But it is probable, that the fixed air ſeparated from fermenting liquors is leſs pure and unmixed than that obtained from chalk, by the addition of oil of vitriol; and that its effects may be varied by the adventitious matters with which it is combined.

THE preſervation of flowers by mephitic air was an event which I little expected, at the commencement of theſe trials: And, as an active mind is ſeldom ſatisfied with the bare obſervance of effects, without inquiring into the cauſes which produce them, I was naturally led into a train of reaſoning on this curious ſubject. It was well known to me, that vegetables, before the putrid fermentation begins, emit a very large proportion of fixed air *(b)*. But this ſeparation can only take place by the mediation of ſome body, which is capable of carrying off what is diſcharged. A wet ſpunge will never become dry in an atmoſphere ſaturated with moiſture; and

(a) MR. HENRY expoſed ſeveral red roſes, in the ſummer of 1774, to a ſtream of pure fixed air, and did not find any change produced in their colour. See his excellent tranſlation of Lavoiſier's Eſſays Phyſical and Chemical, which he has enriched with various uſeful notes, p. 130.

(b) See Prieſtley's Obſervations, vol. I.

 red-hot

red-hot wood ceaſes to burn in inflammable air, which is already loaded with phlogiſton. I was induced, therefore, to ſuppoſe, that the flight of mephitic air from flowers, which ſeems to conſtitute the firſt ſtage of their decay, is prevented, or conſiderably retarded by ſurrounding them with the ſame ſpecies of air, and by excluding from them the common atmoſphere, its proper vehicle.

But the proſecution of my experiments diſcovered to me, that fixed air not only retards the decay, but actually continues the vegetation of plants, and affords them a *pabulum*, which is adequate to the ſupport of life and vigour in them, for a conſiderable length of time.

Tueſday. A sprig of mint was ſuſpended, with the root upwards, in a veſſel of fixed air. The ſucceeding day, it was as freſh and verdant as when firſt gathered. Another ſprig, collected at the ſame time and from the ſame bed, which lay upon my table, was quite withered. Friday, the fourth day, a curve was formed in the middle of the ſtalk, and the top of the ſprig had riſen about an inch, perpendicularly, towards the mouth of the veſſel. Saturday, the mint continued to grow and to aſcend, looking vigorous and freſh: The root, which was very ſmall, appeared quite dry, ſo that the nouriſhment, probably, was imbibed, by the leaves. Tueſday, having

having been abſent two days, the plant was not ſupplied with freſh ſtreams of air: It was ſtill in vigorous vegetation. Friday, the eleventh day of the experiment, the plant was taken out. It was perfectly freſh, but whilſt it lay on my ſtudy table the leaves grew ſoft and flaccid, and in leſs than ſix hours it ſeemed to be withered. The mercury in Fahrenheit's thermometer, during the courſe of this experiment, ſtood from ſixty to ſixty-nine degrees in the ſhade and open air, at two o'clock in the afternoon.

March 23d. Two SPRIGS of MINT with their roots, freſh gathered from the ſame bed, and nearly alike in ſize, were each put into a half ounce phial, filled with rain-water. One of them was ſuſpended, four days and a half, in a veſſel of fixed air, and frequently ſupplied, from chalk and oil of vitriol, with freſh ſtreams of it. The other was placed near it, in the common atmoſphere of my ſtudy: And a few ſprigs of mint, with their roots, were at the ſame time laid upon the table. The latter withered in about twelve hours; and in twenty-four hours were dry and quite ſhriveled. The ſprig in the fixed air flouriſhed greatly; ſhot out freſh leaves from the part immediately above the neck of the phial; expanded its leaves; looked verdant; and, when taken out of the fixed air, had gained, in length, more than half an inch. The ſprig in the common

mon atmoſphere looked ſickly; the leaves were contracted, had a brown and curled appearance, and ſeveral of them were become dead and rotten.

March 28th. The flouriſhing ſprig of mint, which had been ſuſpended in the fixed air, was now placed in the common atmoſphere of my ſtudy; and the other, which was ſo much faded, was put into the veſſel of fixed air. In two hours time, the leaves of the former began to droop and grow flaccid, like a plant taken from a hot-bed; and in twenty-four hours they were in a withered ſtate. The latter ſprig was much revived by the fixed air; but did not vegetate in nearly ſo vigorous a manner as the firſt had done. It was kept four days in the veſſel, and daily furniſhed with freſh ſupplies of fixed air.

April 1ſt. The water, in which the ſprig of mint grew that had been ſuſpended in fixed air, became impregnated with this active principle, as appeared from its acidulous taſte, and from its producing an inſtant precipitation when mixed with lime water. This incited me to try how a plant would vegetate in mephitic water, with its leaves and branches expoſed to the common atmoſphere. A ſprig of mint was, therefore, put into a phial, containing about ſix ounces of it. The ſtalk paſſed through a perpendicular groove, cut in a cork, which ſtopped the mouth

of

of the bottle, to prevent the efcape of the fixed air. In two days, the leaves of the mint became curled at the edges; and the plant feemed to be in a lefs thriving ftate, than another fprig of mint placed in rain-water, which ferved as a ftandard. Sufpecting that the ftalk of the mint was compreffed and injured by the cork, I renewed the experiment, ufing frefh fprigs of mint, and other portions of water; and leaving the mouth of the phial, which held the mephitic water, open to the external air. The vegetation of the plant, in this water, was now very vigorous; and the growth of it, in fix days, confiderably exceeded that of the ftandard.

April 8th. THE experiment of March 23d was repeated; and the fprig of mint, placed in a phial containing half an ounce of rain-water, and fufpended in a veffel conftantly fupplied with frefh ftreams of fixed air, grew above an inch within the fpace of fix days. Another fprig, in half an ounce of fimple rain-water, was in a much lefs healthy ftate, and had fcarcely acquired any perceptible increafe in that time.

April 14th. THIS experiment was repeated with a fprig of BALM, which flourifhed and grew faft in the fixed air.

IT has been fhewn, that a plant grows fafter in mephitic, than in fimple unimpregnated water. The following experiments feem to evince, that the

the fixed air is abſorbed by the roots of the vegetable; and that it affords them real nouriſhment.

April 18th. A SPRIG of MINT, with a ſhort root, was put into a ſix ounce phial, full of rain-water ſtrongly impregnated with fixed air. Another phial of the like ſize was filled with the ſame mephitic water, and placed, without a cork, contiguous to the former, upon a ſhelf in my ſtudy. At the end of four days, they were carefully examined; the ſprig of mint was in a very flouriſhing ſtate, and the water in which it grew had loſt its acidulous taſte; yet it produced a precipitation when mixed with lime water. But the ſtandard of mephitic water ſtill retained a conſiderable degree of pungency; and when poured into lime water rendered it quite milky.

AN AURICULA, full blown, and juſt gathered from my garden at Hart-Hill, was ſuſpended by a ſtring in the veſſel of fixed air, and frequently ſupplied with freſh ſtreams of it. The bloom of this delicate flower continued perfectly unimpaired during eight days, when it was withdrawn, as the proſecution of the experiment interfered with another which I had in view. The auricula, when taken out of the fixed air, withered in a few hours.

May 2d. A LILAC, before the flower was blown, was put into the veſſel of fixed air, and occaſionally, but

but not frequently ſupplied with freſh ſtreams of it. It weighed, at the commencement of this experiment, two ſcruples thirteen grains and a half; and when taken out, at the expiration of ſeven days, only thirty-three grains; having loſt one ſcruple and half a grain of its weight. The flower was a little withered, as much, I conjectured, as it would have been by lying in the open air about ſix hours. The ſtalk was dry. This flower was without any green leaves; and it is not improbable, that the abſorbent veſſels are confined to theſe leaves *(d)*.

A TULIP, about half blown, was put into the veſſel with the lilac. It ſeemed not to flouriſh, but opened ſo much in the veſſel, that, at the end of ſeven days, I found a difficulty in taking it out of the aperture, through which at firſt it had paſſed very readily. The tulip had no leaves: Its colour remained unchanged.

May 10th. A BRANCH of LILAC, which weighed eighty-ſix grains and a half, was put into the veſſel. Some of the flowers were blown; but moſt of them remained in a cloſed ſtate. I plucked off four green leaves, before the branch was expoſed to the fixed air, to ſee whether it would grow and flouriſh by the abſorption of the flowers and ſtalk alone. It ſhould be re-

(d) SEE Grew's Anatomy of Plants. Hale's Statical Eſſays Hunter's Georgical Eſſays.

marked

marked, that the ſtalk of the lilac is woody and not very ſucculent.

May 18th. THE air had not been renewed during forty-eight hours, owing to my abſence from Mancheſter. Several of the flower cups of the lilac were more open than at firſt; but the flowers were ſomewhat withered, probably as much as they would have been by lying eight or ten hours in the open air. The whole branch had loſt eighteen grains of its weight.

A PURPLE FLOWER, unblown, was ſuſpended in the veſſel with the lilac. It weighed two ſcruples and ten grains, and was without leaves. The ſtalk was ſucculent.

May 18th. THE air had not been renewed during forty-eight hours, yet the flower was perfectly freſh, and its purple colour remained unchanged. Several of the flower cups were opened, and the ſeeds diſplayed. It had loſt ſix grains of its weight.

HAVING thus opened a path into a new and fertile region of ſcience, I ſhall diſcontinue my reſearches for a while, with a reſolution however to reſume them in the ſpring of the ſucceeding year. In the mean time, I ſhall think myſelf happy if I can prevail upon my philoſophical friends to engage in the ſame purſuit, by offering them, as a clue, theſe few experiments; together with the following obſervations and conjectures, which

8. As fixed air is ſo favourable to the growth of vegetables, perhaps it may equally contribute to the nouriſhment and ſupport of animals. It is ſeparated from our food, during the proceſs of digeſtion; and it may only be injurious to us when too copious; as exceſs in the quantity of water proves hurtful to the roots of plants.

N. B. It may be proper to inform the reader, who would chooſe to repeat my experiments, that they were generally made with Dr. Nooth's apparatus for impregnating water with fixed air.

May 20, 1775.

ADDITIONAL OBSERVATIONS

ON THE EFFECTS OF FIXED AIR,

IN

PROMOTING THE GROWTH OF PLANTS.

I HAVE communicated to many of my friends an account of the experiments, which I made in the ſpring of 1775, on vegetation, as influenced by fixed air. And I flatter myſelf, that the ſubject will engage the attention, and excite the trials of thoſe, who have a taſte for purſuits of this nature. Mr. Bew, who was a witneſs to the flouriſhing ſtate of my ſprigs of mint, growing in mephitic water, has lately tried a ſimilar experiment with two hyacinths. And I ſhall lay before the reader his account of the ſucceſs of it.

"December 2, 1775. Two hyacinth bulbs, " each weighing four drachms and a few grains, " were placed in glaſſes made for the purpoſe " of vegetating bulbous roots. One glaſs was " ſupplied with ſeven ounces and a half of pump- " water, impregnated with fixed air; the other " with the ſame quantity of rain-water.

"NEITHER of the plants had made much " progreſs in vegetation. Some white fibrous " roots were ſhooting from the plant ſupplied with " rain water, but none from that which had the " water with fixed air.

"December 17th. SEVERAL beautiful white " fibres were diſcovered, ſhooting from the root " ſupplied with fixed air; and both plants were " beginning to vegetate.

"THE bulb ſupplied with rain-water ſeemed, " at firſt, to make the greater progreſs in vege- " tation. The fibrous roots of the other were, " however, much ſtronger, whiter, and more " tranſparent.

" They were conſtantly ſupplied with their " reſpective kinds of water; and, at intervals, " when I concluded that the factitious air was " exhauſted by the plant, the whole was poured " off; and each glaſs filled, at the ſame time, " with the ſame quantity of its proper water.

" January 1, 1776. The plant immerſed in " the water impregnated with fixed air, ſurpaſſed " the other in the ſtrength and colour of its " leaves, which were of a lively green, and the " roots of a moſt beautiful tranſparent white. " The other plant, though apparently healthy, " had very few roots.

" January 16th. Both plants continued to " vegetate, but the one ſupplied with fixed air " much more than the other. And it ſeemed " equally forward with ſome other bulbs, which " had been placed in common rain-water, nearly " a month before. An accident, however, hap- " pened at this time, which, I apprehended, " would have put an end to my experiment. " My ſervant, in letting down a large curtain " before the window where the glaſſes were " placed, overturned that which contained the " water with fixed air. The night was rather " ſevere, and the plant lay ten or eleven hours " out of water. I replaced it in another glaſs " with the mephitic water, and continued to " ſupply them as uſual.

"January 21ſt. I WAS much ſurprized to "find the plant had recovered its former vigour, "and was advancing a ſtem with buds for "flowering, which the other plant ſhewed no "ſigns of.

"THE weather at this time became ſo cold, "that I thought it neceſſary to remove all the "plants out of the window of my parlour to a "warmer part of the room, that the progreſs of "their vegetation might not be retarded.

"February 6th. THE glaſſes were replaced "in the window, and each ſeemed in a very "healthy ſtate. That, ſupplied with mephitic "water, viſibly increaſed every day.

"THE plant in the rain-water had advanced "a ſtem with buds; but not more than half "the ſize of the other.

"February 27th. THE hyacinth, which had "been ſupplied with water impregnated with "fixed air, was in full blow, appeared remark-"ably ſtrong, and diffuſed the delicate fragrance "peculiar to the flower. It meaſured, from the "bulb, full ſixteen inches. I withdrew it gently "from the water, and found it weighed two "ounces, two drachms, and five grains.

"THE other hyacinth was juſt beginning to "expand its flower. It meaſured no more than "ten inches from the bulb; and, though freſh "vigorous, weighed only one ounce, one drachm, "and ſix grains."

THIS

This experiment of Mr. Bew would have been more decisive, if he had employed rain-water impregnated with fixed air, and not pump-water. But it coincides with the trials which I have related, and sufficiently evinces the powerful influence of this principle on vegetation.

It is a common custom with gardeners to expose pump-water to the sun and air, to soften it, many hours before they use it for the purpose of sprinkling their plants and flowers. This should seem to be an injudicious practice, if the hardness of the water arise, as it often does, from the fixed air which it contains. For it will thus be deprived of that constituent part, which has been shewn to be so friendly to vegetable life. Mephitic air is found in many common springs; and such should always be selected for the uses of gardening and agriculture. In green houses, water artificially impregnated might be employed, without any great trouble or expence.

Dr. Priestley, whose accuracy and fidelity are not less distinguished than his learning and ingenuity, having drawn conclusions, from the prosecution of this subject, concerning the influence of fixed air on vegetation, which militate totally with mine; I refumed the inquiry, and engaged feveral of my friends in it. The refult of all our trials was uniformly the fame as before, viz. that fixed air, in a due proportion, is fo favourable to vegetable growth, that it may juftly be deemed a *pabulum* of plants. Dr. Prieftley's fubfequent experiments, however, were ftill contradictory to mine: And in one of his very friendly letters to me, he thus expreffes himfelf. "In all thefe "cafes, you will fay, I choke the plants with "too great a quantity of *wholefome* nourifhment: "And to all yours I fay, you do not give them "enough of the *noxious matter* to kill them. "Thus the amicable controverfy muft reft be-"tween us; and, like all other combatants, we "fhall both fing Te Deum." But I felt little difpofition to exultation on fuch an occafion, and dropt the fubject, confcious that, though nature is always the fame, we often view her under fallacious appearances. Time, however, and the refearches of foreign philofophers have thrown new lights on this difputed point. And I am informed, by a letter from our common friend, Mr. Vaughan, that Dr. Prieftley now admits the falubrity of fixed air to vegetable life. I fhall copy the paragraph, which contains the account. "Dr. Prieftley tells me "of a very valuable book, written by a perfon "at Geneva, on vegetation; particularly as to "the

"the influence of light, which he maintains to "be a phlogiſticating proceſs, acting on the re-"ſinous parts of plants only. He alſo affirms, to "the ſatisfaction of Dr. Prieſtley, that not only "phlogiſton is the grand *pabulum* of plants, "but that its predominant form of reception is "that of fixed air; which, in a proper degree "and place of application, he ſhews to be ſalu-"tary to all plants whatever" *(g)*.

In a ſubſequent paper of the ſame work, Mr. Henry has addreſſed to me, OBSERVATIONS *on the* INFLUENCE *of* FIXED AIR *on* VEGETATION; *and on the* PROBABLE CAUSE *of the* DIFFERENCE *in the* RESULTS *of* VARIOUS EXPERIMENTS *made on that* SUBJECT; from which I ſhall take the liberty of making the following extracts.

"It is now many years ſince, from ſome "experiments which you had made on the effects "of fixed air, applied to the leaves and roots of "plants, you, as appeared to me at that time, "*juſtly* concluded, that fixed air affords a *pabu-*"*lum* for plants, which is equal to the ſupport "of their life and vigour, for a conſiderable time. "Some of theſe experiments were ſeemingly "contradictory to the reſults of thoſe related by "Dr. Prieſtley in his firſt volume. The doctor "therefore requeſted, that you or I would repeat "them in veſſels containing *pure* fixed air. For

(g) See the Memoirs of the Mancheſter Philoſophical Society, vol. II. p. 330.

"the

" the doctor had found, that plants confined in " *pure* fixed air perished sooner than in com- " mon air.

" I all along understood your meaning to be, " not that fixed air, in a pure state, and quite " stagnant, was nutritive to plants; but, that gra- " dually applied, and in a continued stream, while " the plant, at the same time, is not confined from " the common air, (in a manner analogous to " what may probably take place in nature) " plants do receive such a portion of nutriment, " from the fixed air, as is sufficient for their " temporary support, even when removed from " every other means of receiving their food. " This, at least, was the idea which I always en- " tertained; and the conclusion to be drawn " from this theory is, that, probably, fixed air " constitutes a part of the food of plants, when " growing in their proper element; such air be- " ing discharged by the different manures, which " are mixed with their native soil; and this " theory, if just, may lead to considerable im- " provements in agriculture. In the third vo- " lume of Experiments and Observations on " different Kinds of Air, Dr. Priestley, at the " same time that he acknowledges, that ' he " could conceive nothing more fair and deci- " sive than your experiments,' declares himself " convinced, that there must have been some

" fallacy

" ſallacy in them; and he ſeems to think, that he " had detected it in two inſtances. The firſt ſup- " poſed cauſe of error was, that your ſtandard " plants, had not been placed in ſimilar veſſels " to thoſe which had been expoſed to the fixed " air: And the other, that, as your experi- " ments were made in Nooth's machine, and as " you had not aſcertained the proportion of fixed " air which was contained in your veſſel, it was " probably, much ſmaller than you had imagined.

" In regard to the animal body, it would ſurely " be wrong to ſay, that nothing is nutritious " or ſalutary to it, but what it could bear to " receive unmixed or undiluted. Why then may " we not ſuppoſe, that though fixed air, when " pure, may be fatal to plants confined in it, " and excluded from free communication with " the common air; yet when applied in proper " doſe, and to plants enjoying a free intercourſe " with the atmoſphere, it may have a contrary " effect, and ſerve to nouriſh and ſupport them?

" But in Dr. Prieſtley's experiments, this *free* " *intercourſe* does not appear to have been allow- " ed; and herein, I apprehend, conſiſted the " cauſe of the difference in our reſults.

" At that time, the conſtitution of fixed air " was not underſtood. It is now, *generally*, " allowed to be formed by a combination of " phlogiſton with the pure part of atmoſpheric

" air.

" air. The firſt of theſe ingredients has been " proved, by the experiments of Dr. Prieſtley and " others, to be favourable to vegetation, while " plants droop and decay when expoſed to the " action of the latter. It ſhould further appear, " from Dr. Ingenhouz's train of experiments, " that plants have the power of ſeparating phlo- " giſton from common air; applying it to their " nurture; and throwing out the pure or de- " phlogiſticated reſiduum, as excrementitious. " Now allowing, what appears highly probable, " that they have a ſimilar power of decompoſing " *fixed air*, and of applying and rejecting its con- " ſtituent parts, our method of conducting the " experiments was *not* injurious to the proceſs; " whereas, when confined in cloſe veſſels, as by " Dr. Prieſtley, the plants would be ſuffocated, " in a manner reverſed to what would happen " to an animal. For, as in that caſe, from a " want of communication with the atmoſphere, " as neceſſary to carry off the phlogiſton thrown " out from the lungs, (according to the beauti- " ful theory of reſpiration advanced, and ſo well " ſupported by Dr. Prieſtley) the animal muſt " periſh; ſo, in the other inſtance, the plant " would die, if cut off from the air of the at- " moſphere, in ſuch manner, that the pure air, " excreted by its veſſels, could not be conveyed " from it. For, in theſe circumſtances, this fluid,

" ſo

" ſo ſalutary to animal, but deſtructive to vegeta-" ble life, muſt be accumulated in the body of the " plant; and, its functions being thus impeded, " death is the neceſſary conſequence.

" This reaſoning ſeems to be confirmed by " ſome of the facts which you have communi-" cated to me, from your Journal. For it ap-" pears, from ſeveral of your experiments, that, " during ſeven hours of the day, viz. from 10, " A. M. to 5, P. M. the plants you employed " were expoſed to varying proportions of fixed " air, ſeldom exceeding $\frac{1}{2}$ the proportion of air, " contained in the veſſel, and never leſs than " $\frac{1}{4}$. But, from 5 o'clock in the evening till " 10 the ſucceeding day, the quantity of fixed " air ſeems to have varied, from $\frac{1}{2}$ to $\frac{1}{17}$ of the " whole air. Now a plant expoſed to ſuch diver-" ſified proportions of air, paſſing too in a ſtream " through the veſſel, muſt be in a favourable " ſtate, both for exhalation, and conſequently " for the proceſs of inhalation alſo" *(b)*.

(b) Memoirs of the Mancheſter Society, vol. II. p. 341—343, 347—349.

ESSAY

ESSAY VII.

MISCELLANEOUS OBSERVATIONS

CONCERNING THE

ACTION OF DIFFERENT

MANURES (*a*).

1. I APPREHEND, that oily ſubſtances cannot produce any conſiderable effect on land, unleſs they be previouſly combined with mucilages, or converted into ſoap, by means of quicklime or fixed alkalis. In this ſtate they meliorate the ſoil in ſeveral ways, viz. by affording a laſting *pabulum* for plants; by fitting it to receive, and preventing the too ſpeedy evaporation of the dews and rains; and by preſenting the food of vegetables, in a due proportion, to the abſorbent veſſels of their roots.

2. SALINE ſubſtances, as they are ſoluble in water, and capable of admiſſion into the vaſcular

(*a*) Inſerted in Dr. Hunter's Georgical Eſſays, p. 486.

tubes

tubes of plants, act more immediately on the earth. Whether they afford any real nutriment to vegetables, or whether their operation depends upon a stimulating power, by which they quicken vegetation, I am at a loss to determine. For that plants are endued with *irritability* is evident from various facts. The sensitive tribe of vegetables afford ocular demonstration of it; and electricity is well known to accelerate the growth of plants, by promoting the ascent of their juices.

3. Common Salt is universally esteemed an excellent manure; but I think it would be still more powerful, if a proper quantity of Epsom salt were added to it. By this combination it would more exactly resemble sea-water, which amazingly fertilizes the marshes over which it flows. The grass of such marshes is purgative to horses and to cattle; which affords a presumptive proof, that sea-salt, mixed with the bittern, may be received into the vessels of plants, in a much larger proportion than when purified and refined. The combination here recommended, will act as a powerful septic, when mixed with the corrupted vegetables, and other putrefying substances on the surface of the earth; and, by this fermentation, will improve the soil.

4. Quicklime is not classed by the modern chemists amongst the salts, though it has some

properties

properties in common with them. It may aɕt, as a manure, by combining with and dividing the particles of clay, and, thus, forming a ſpecies of marl; by uniting with the oily ſubſtances contained in the ſoil, and rendering them ſoluble in water; and by abſorbing the dews and rains, and preventing them from ſinking too ſpeedily into the earth, by which the food of plants is waſhed from their radical fibres.

5. LIME and the fixed alkalis are more powerful agents, than neutral ſalts, in preparing the food of vegetables, by their operation on the oils and mucilages which exiſt in the ſoil, and which have been ſupplied by manures, or derived from the atmoſphere.

AUGUST 20, 1770.

ESSAY VIII.

REMARKS

ON DIFFERENT

ABSORBENTS.

LANGIUS and Homberg, two able chemiſts, have attempted to aſcertain the comparative powers of various abſorbents. But the acids which they employed being of the mineral claſs, and totally different from thoſe which exiſt in the human body, no accurate concluſions can be drawn from their trials, concerning the medicinal action of ſuch abſorbents *(a)*. The following table exhibits the reſult of ſome experiments, which I made, about two years ago (February 1774), on this ſubject.

TABLE.

Abſorbents.	Diſtilled Water.	Drops of White Wine Vinegar.
Ten grains of Earth of Alum,	- half an ounce,	13.
Magneſia,	- - - -	24.

(a) See Lewis's new Diſpenſatory, p. 64.

 Calcined

Abſorbents.	Diſtilled Water.	Drops of White Wine Vinegar.
Calcined Magneſia,	- - -	42.
Prepared Chalk,	- - -	14.
Compound Powder of Crabs Claws,	-	10.
Salt of Tartar,	- - -	90.
Volatile Sal Ammoniac,	- - -	110.
Ten drops of Lixivium Tartari,	- -	50.
Spirits of Hartſhorn,	- - -	45.

There is ſuch a diverſity in the purity of the ſame ſpecies of abſorbents, as well as in the ſtrength of different vinegars, that I am ſenſible theſe experiments are vague and indeterminate; though they were made with much attention, and the drops of acid here ſet down, were the medium quantity of ſeveral trials. However, as the ſubject admits not, ſo neither does it require mathematical certainty. And we may, with ſafety and advantage, in this, as we are obliged to do in many other inſtances, found both our reaſoning and practice on *data*, which approach nearly to truth.

The method which I purſued in making the experiments, from which the foregoing table is deduced, was to add ſix or eight drops of the acid to the abſorbent; then to pour half an ounce of diſtilled water upon it; and afterwards to inſtil, *guttatim*, as much vinegar as barely to occaſion a perceptible prevalence of the acid. In ſuch combinations

combinations, the continuance of the effervefcence is no teft, that faturation has not taken place. Three hundred drops of white wine vinegar were added, in the way above defcribed, to ten grains of volatile fal ammoniac. Every additional drop ftill produced air bubbles; by which appearance I was fo much deceived, that I fhould have continued to add more vinegar, had I not found, by tafting the mixture, that it was extremely four. And when I put into it a few grains of the volatile falt, a very brifk effervefcence enfued. From this trial it fhould feem, that the particles of the alkali combine with the acid more flowly and gradually than is commonly fuppofed; and this obfervation will be found to merit the attention of apothecaries.

THE combination of vinegar, or juice of lemons, with *lixivium tartari* yielded very little fixed air in my experiments. This mixture, therefore, is not well adapted to be given in the act of effervefcence.

THE mixtures of vinegar and earth of alum, alfo, emitted very few air bubbles. But the fame acid with chalk, or compound powder of crab's claws, fwelled much, and effervefced violently.

THE earth of alum, which I employed in thefe experiments, was prepared in the following manner. Two pounds of roch alum, freed, by washing, from all external impurities, were dissolved in about five gallons of soft water. To this liquor, whilst hot, four pounds and a half of a filtered solution of pot-ashes were gradually added. The precipitated earth was repeatedly washed, in hot and cold water, till it was entirely divested of saltness; and afterwards placed upon chalk stones, to be thoroughly dried. The alum, reduced to this state, weighed only four ounces, six drachms, and twelve grains.

At the time when I was engaged in these inquiries, I received from a gentleman, just returned from Jamaica, a quantity of the essential salt of lemons, which he had made himself, by evaporating, in the sun, the juice of that fruit, till it assumed a crystallized form. This acid was very grateful to the palate; and I dissolved such a quantity of it in distilled water, as to produce a liquor nearly resembling fresh lemon juice. One scruple of it, as exactly as I could judge, seemed to be equal to a lemon of a common size.

An ounce phial, filled to the brim with the acid liquor thus made, weighed two ounces, five drachms, and half a grain. But an equal quantity of a saturated solution of the earth of alum in the same liquor, after being carefully filtered, weighed eight grains heavier; and a like solution of of pure magneſia*(b)* twelve grains and a half. From hence it appears, that magneſia is much more ſoluble in the vegetable acid, than the earth of alum. But the liquor is extremely nauſeous to the taſte; whereas the ſolution of the earth of alum is not unpleaſant, having a ſlight degree of ſweetneſs and ſtypticity.

As the ſenſible qualities of alum, and of its earth, in combination with the vegetable acid, ſo nearly reſemble each other, we may preſume, that they are ſimilar in their medicinal powers. And I have employed this abſorbent with conſiderable advantage, in ſuch caſes of acidity as ariſe from an *atonia* of the ſtomach and inteſtines. But we ſometimes obſerve, that the ſame diſordered ſtate of the bowels generates an acid in the ſtomach and *duodenum*, and a highly putrid acrimony in the lower inteſtines. A gentleman, after a moderate dinner of chicken, and a ſupper of apple tart and new milk, was affected, in the night-time, with great flatulency. His diſcharges of wind upwards were attended with the moſt corroſive acidity; thoſe downwards were uncommonly putrid and noiſome. His complaints terminated in a *diarrhœa*; and his evacuations were hot, ſharp, and intolerably fœtid. A lady had a rheumatic fever, about the middle of laſt

(b) The magneſia I had from Mr. Henry, who is well known to prepare it with great ſkill and attention.

ſummer, which, towards the concluſion, aſſumed a putrid type. Her ſtools were frequent and very offenſive; and ſhe had the moſt black and aphthous tongue I ever ſaw. Clyſters of fixed air were injected; acids, vegetable and mineral, were freely adminiſtered; and by theſe, and other means, the *diarrhœa* was reſtrained. A ſudden change took place in the ſtate of her bowels; and an acid acrimony ſeemed now to prevail as much as the putrid one had done before. In ſuch caſes as theſe, an intelligent phyſician will conſider chalk, crab's eyes, and other ſeptic earths, as contraindicated; and will be glad to avail himſelf of ſuch an abſorbent as will, at the ſame time, corroborate and reſiſt putrefaction. The earth of alum might be deemed, *à priori*, to poſſeſs theſe powers, in a very conſiderable degree; but, from experiments, I find, that, even when combined with the vegetable acid, it is a very weak antiſeptic. I ſaturated an ounce of lemon juice with it; another ounce with pure magneſia; and a third with *lixivium tartari*; and then added to each half an ounce of raw mutton, chopped very ſmall. The phials containing the mixtures were ſlightly corked, and placed in a heat of about a hundred degrees of Fahrenheit's ſcale. A fourth phial, which was intended for a ſtandard, contained the ſame quantity of mutton, and an ounce of diſtilled water. In twenty-one hours,

hours, the mixture with the earth of alum was in briſk fermentation; the liquor was of a brown colour; much froth was collected on the ſurface, and it ſmelled offenſively, like faded cheeſe.

The mixture with magneſia did not ferment much; the liquor was of a bloody colour, and had a very offenſive and putrid ſmell.

The ſaline mixture was perfectly ſweet, and had undergone only a ſlight fermentation.

The ſtandard was extremely putrid, and the liquor very bloody.

In forty-eight hours, the aluminous mixture was more putrid and offenſive than that which contained the magneſia. The ſaline mixture continued perfectly ſweet.

I varied this experiment afterwards, by leaving the vegetable acid out of the mixtures; and uſing only the earth of alum, chalk, and magneſia. They all powerfully accelerated the corruption of the fleſh; the earth of alum proving the moſt, and magneſia the leaſt ſeptic.

A very ingenious chemiſt has lately propoſed to the trial of the faculty a new ſaline preparation, namely, the vegetable alkali diſſolved in water, and perfectly ſaturated with fixed air, which he has ſhewn to be an acid *(c)*. This compound

(c) See Mr. Bewly's excellent Letters, in the Appendix to Dr. Prieſtley's ſecond Volume of Obſervations on various kinds of Air.

he recommends, as a febrifuge and antiseptic, in fevers, and other disorders of a putrid tendency. I was so much pleased with the idea of this neutral julep, that I immediately prepared a small quantity of it, by mixing ten drachms of the *lixivium tartari* with about a quart of pure water, and strongly impregnating the solution with fixed air, by means of Dr. Nooth's apparatus. The nauseous flavour of the alkali is almost entirely corrected by this process, and the liquor has a grateful and acidulous taste. The *lixivium tartari* seems to attract a very considerable quantity of fixed air *(d)*; and, as the mephitic acid has a weaker relation to it than any other, it will be separated in the stomach; and this elegant saline julep will, thus, produce the good effects of a tonic and absorbent. But, when it is thought expedient to give this julep in a large quantity, not more than a drachm of *lixivium tartari* should be added to each pint of water. And, even in this proportion, the alkali may prove too diuretic, except in dropsical cases, to which it seems to be well adapted. The pleasantest beverage I have yet been able to prepare,

(d) THIS will appear very evident by comparing together the effervescence produced in the neutralized and unneutralized *lixivium tartari*, when the vitriolic acid is added to equal quantities of each of them.

is

is made by diſſolving a drachm and a half of the foſſil alkali, and twenty-five grains of bay ſalt, in three pints of pure water, which is then to be ſtrongly impregnated with fixed air. This liquor exactly reſembles very good Seltzer water; and may be drunk to ſatiety in hot climates in hectic, inflammatory, or putrid diſorders, without danger, and with great advantage.

ESSAY IX.

ON THE

INTERNAL REGULATION

OF

HOSPITALS.

ADDRESSED TO MR. AIKIN.*

MANCHESTER, OCTOBER 1, 1771.

I HAVE perufed with great pleafure your ingenious THOUGHTS ON HOSPITALS. The importance of the fubject, and the judicious manner in which you have treated it, cannot fail to excite the attention, and to fecure to you the approbation of the public. It is a melancholy confideration, that thefe charitable inftitutions, which are intended for the health and prefervation of mankind, may too often be ranked amongft the caufes of ficknefs and mortality *(a)*. This obfervation

* Inferted at the end of AIKIN's *Thoughts on Hofpitals*.

(a) A THIRD of all who die at Paris, die in hofpitals. In the *Hôtel-Dieu*, a great hofpital fituated in the middle of that city, we behold a horrid fcene of mifery; for, the beds being

obſervation you have well illuſtrated, by pointing out the pernicious effects of tainted air; the falſe œconomy of crowding a number of ſick perſons into as little ſpace as poſſible; and the miſtaken humanity of admitting patients, who labour under diſeaſes which are contagious in their nature, incapable of relief, or liable to be aggravated by confinement in an impure atmoſphere.

But as ſo many infirmaries are erected in different parts of the kingdom, on plans which cannot now be altered; and as they are governed by

being too few for the numbers admitted, it is common to ſee four, ſix, or even eight patients in a bed together, lying four at one end, and four at the other. The number annually admitted into this hoſpital amounts to nearly twenty-two thouſand; (vid. Police of France, p. 83) and I am well informed, that *two* in *nine*, of all received from 1724 to 1763, have died. In the two great hoſpitals of London, St. Thomas's and St. Bartholomew's, about ſix hundred die annually, or *one* in *thirteen* of all admitted as in-patients. Vid. Price on the Expectation of Lives, p. 216. In the Northampton infirmary, *one* in *nineteen* of the in-patients (*communibus annis*) dies every year; and in that of Mancheſter, which is built in an airy ſituation, and tolerably well ventilated, *one* in *twenty-two*. This proportion of deaths, I apprehend, exceeds the mortality which occurs in private practice: And it will appear to be more conſiderable, when we recollect, that, beſides the patients who are diſmiſſed as incurable, improper objects, or on account of irregularity; the event of whoſe caſes remains unknown, the ſmall-pox, meaſles, *lues venerea*, fevers, and other dangerous and fatal diſtempers, are excluded from admiſſion into theſe hoſpitals.

by eſtabliſhed laws, which, however erroneous, will ſtill, from the force of cuſtom, continue to be obſerved, it were to be wiſhed, that ſome means could be deviſed of obviating the inconveniences which ariſe from their preſent conſtruction, as well as mode of regulation. Permit me to ſuggeſt to you a few hints on this ſubject, which I ſhall hope to ſee improved and enlarged, if they fall within the deſign of your uſeful publication.

AIR, DIET and MEDICINE, are the three great agents to be employed, in preventing and correcting putrefaction and contagion in hoſpitals. A gallon of air is conſumed every minute by a man in health; a ſick perſon requires a larger ſupply, becauſe he more quickly contaminates it; and it is obſerved, that animals expire ſooner in foul air, than *in vacuo*. Beſides ventilators, therefore, and ſaſhes ſliding downwards ſo as to open at top, apertures ſhould be made in the wall, oppoſite to the windows, correſponding to them in number, and of ſufficient dimenſions. This is an improvement lately adopted in the infirmary at Leiceſter, and has been found to ſucceed. The larger wards ſhould have a fire-place at each end of them; and, in ſummer time, the diſcharge of foul air, by the pipes of the chimney, may be continued by means of a flue, communicating with a fire below. I ſhould not omit to mention, that the ſalubrity of the air is very much influenced by its temperature, which ought to be regulated by a thermometer, placed in the centre of every room.

But ſupplies of the pureſt air are inſufficient to deſtroy contagion; of which I could produce ſeveral undeniable proofs, from the beſt authority. It is neceſſary, therefore, to correct the noxious effluvia which ariſe from ſo many diſtempered bodies, afflicted perhaps with mortifications, carious bones, malignant ulcers, or putrid fevers. This I apprehend may be effected by ſprinkling, or rather waſhing, daily, the apartments of the ſick with vinegar and an infuſion of deal ſaw-duſt, or with oil of vitriol and water; by frequently fumigating them with the ſteams of boiling vinegar and tar, or, if diſeaſes of extraordinary malignancy occur, with boiling vinegar, myrrh, and camphor; by uſing wood fuel, particularly fir, and occaſionally dipping the faggots in tar; by ventilating the bed clothes of ſuch patients as are able to ſit up or walk about, and afterwards impregnating them with the antiſeptic vapours above-mentioned; and by obliging the ſick to conform ſtrictly to the rules of nicety and cleanlineſs. If any of them have been accuſtomed to ſmoking, they ſhould be allowed pipes and tobacco, when ſuch an indulgence will not be injurious. The patients ſhould have their

their linen very frequently renewed; and their ſhirts and ſheets ſhould be fumigated with frankincenſe, before they are uſed. The dreſſings of foul ulcers, &c. as ſoon as they are removed, ſhould be thrown into veſſels of vinegar, or of oil of vitriol and water, and carried out of the wards with all convenient expedition. It is to be wiſhed, that ſalves were baniſhed from hoſpital practice; and I rejoice, that, in a former work, you have ſo ſtrongly expreſſed your diſapprobation of them *(b)*. Oil, by heat, acquires a rancidity which renders it both ſtimulant and ſeptic; and, by theſe qualities, it increaſes the acrimony and fœtor of all purulent diſcharges. Poultices either of carrots or white bread, or tow lightly ſpread over with the mucilage of ſtarch, mixed with ſuch a proportion of neatsfoot oil as to prevent its growing ſtiff, might perhaps be uſefully ſubſtituted, as ſoft defenſatives, in the room of plaſters and cerates. Twelve parts of the mucilage, and one of oil mix uniformly together without heat, are of a due conſiſtence, and continue moiſt a ſufficient length of time. In ſome caſes, it may be of advantage, to prepare the mucilage of ſtarch with the ſaturnine water of Goulard; which, with the neatsfoot oil, will furniſh an emollient, antiſeptic, and

(b) Obſervations on the External Uſe of preparations of Lead.

moderately

moderately aſtringent topic, much ſuperior, I apprehend, to the *unguentum tripharmacum*.

NEXT to the ſalubrity of the AIR, a well-regulated DIET may be conſidered as the moſt powerful preſervative againſt the in-bred diſeaſes of hoſpitals. In ſummer and autumn, when putrid diſtempers are moſt prevalent, the patients ſhould be liberally ſupplied with fruit. Nor will the procuring of it be attended either with difficulty or expence, if it be intimated to the patrons of theſe charities, and to other well-diſpoſed perſons, that ſuch donations will be highly acceptable.

RICE forms a conſiderable article in the table of diet, of almoſt every infirmary. But, as a wholeſome aliment, it is much inferior to ſalep, which I believe is ſeldom, if ever uſed. I digeſted ſeveral mixtures, prepared of mutton and water, beat up with bread, ſea biſcuit, ſalep, rice flour, ſago powder, potatoe, old cheeſe, &c. in a heat equal to that of the human body. In forty-eight hours, they had all acquired a vinous ſmell, and were in briſk fermentation, except the mixture with rice, which did not emit many air bubbles, and was but little changed. The third day, ſome of the mixtures were ſweet, and continued to ferment; others had loſt their inteſtine motion, and were ſour; but the one which contained the rice was become putrid. From this experiment it appears, that rice, as an aliment,

aliment, is ſlow of fermentation, and a very weak corrector of putrefaction: It is therefore an improper diet for hoſpital patients. Nor can it be conſidered as a very nutritive kind of food, on account of its difficult ſolubility in the ſtomach. Experience confirms the truth of this concluſion; for it is obſerved, by the planters in the Weſt Indies, that the negroes grow thin, and are leſs able to work, whilſt they ſubſiſt upon rice.

SALEP is ſaid to contain the greateſt quantity of vegetable nouriſhment under the ſmalleſt bulk; and from its reſtorative, mucilaginous, and demulcent qualities, it deſerves to be conſidered as a *medicinal diet*. It obtunds the acrimony of the fluids, and, at the ſame time, is eaſily aſſimilated into a mild and wholeſome chyle. In diarrhœas, and in the dyſentery, it is highly ſerviceable, by ſheathing the internal coat of the inteſtines, by abating irritation, and gently correcting putrefaction. In the ſymptomatic fever, which ariſes from the abſorption of pus, from ulcers in the lungs, from wounds, or from amputation, ſalep uſed plentifully, is an admirable demulcent *(c)*.

CHEESE, I apprehend, is an unwholeſome diet for convaleſcents, becauſe, when new, it is almoſt

(c) See vol. I. p. 289, 292.

indigeſtible; and although, when mellowed by age, I have obſerved, that it ferments readily with fleſh and water, yet it ſeparates a rancid oil, which ſeems incapable of any further change, and, as a ſeptic, muſt be pernicious. For hoſpital patients are ſo liable to relapſes, that the ſlighteſt error of diet may occaſion them. The infuſion of malt, which is ſtrongly recommended in the ſcurvy at ſea, may perhaps, as an antiſeptic, be no leſs uſeful in hoſpitals. It may be allowed the patients for common drink, in lieu of table beer, which, having undergone the vinous fermentation, has loſt, in ſome meaſure, the power of correcting or ſweetening putrefaction. Should this liquor prove too aperient, a few red roſe leaves, or balauſtines, infuſed with the malt, will obviate this effect, without communicating any diſagreeable flavour. The flour of malt might alſo be employed for making gruel, milk pottage, or puddings.

With reſpect to animal food, all ſalted and ſmoke-dried meats are, I believe, generally diſallowed. Pork ſhould likewiſe be forbidden, as it is the moſt putreſcent kind of fleſh, and tends to diminiſh perſpiration. Care ſhould be taken alſo, that the meat, which is killed for the uſe of infirmaries, be more than uſually blooded, that it may not, by becoming ſoon tainted, concur,

 with

with other unavoidable caufes, in the production of putrid difeafes.

Concerning medicines little more can be fuggefted, than that, in prefcribing them, regard fhould be had not only to the prefent fymptoms, but alfo to the putrid tendency, and contagious nature of hofpital difeafes. And, as the courfe of infection is ufually flow, the phyfician fhould carefully watch its firft acceffion; and, by fuitable remedies, inftantly check its progrefs.—In malignant fevers, befides adminiftering the Peruvian bark in fubftance or decoction, a light infufion of it, well acidulated, may be directed for the common drink of the patient. But, in lefs urgent cafes, vinegar, or cream of tartar whey will be a more grateful diluent, and fufficiently antifeptic. It would be a farther means of correcting putrefaction, and would anfwer other ufeful purpofes, if the fick were to wafh their faces, and bathe their feet and hands, every morning and evening, in a decoction of bark, or of chamomile flowers, mixed with vinegar.

I have thus, my dear friend, very imperfectly drawn the outlines of a plan for rendering hofpitals, upon their prefent eftablifhment, more falutary to the fick, and confequently more ufeful to the public; and I flatter myfelf you will improve and finifh it. Permit me, before I conclude, to mention an ingenious contrivance, ufed

in

in the infirmary at Leicester, which contributes greatly to the ease and convenience of the patients. The bedsteads, which are of iron painted, are so made, that the backs, by means of a screw, may be raised or lowered, with the greatest facility. This improvement was suggested by Dr. Vaughan; and executed, under the direction of Dr. Ash, at Birmingham.

MISCELLANEOUS

OBSERVATIONS,

CASES, AND INQUIRIES.

FATAL EFFECTS OF YEW LEAVES.

ON Friday, March 25th, 1774, three children of James Buckley, a labouring man at Longſight, near Mancheſter, were killed by taking a ſmall quantity of the freſh leaves of the yew tree, or *taxus officinalis* of Caſpar Bauhin *(a)*. The oldeſt child was five, the ſecond four, and the youngeſt three years of age. They were all ſuppoſed to be affected with worms; and this poiſon was given them, by the recommendation of ſome ignorant perſon, as a powerful remedy for that diſorder. The *dried leaves* were firſt employed; and a ſpoonful of them, mixed with brown ſugar, was divided into three equal doſes, which the children took at ſeven o'clock in the morning. At eight, they had each a meſs

(a) Taxus baccata Lin.

of

of pottage, prepared of butter-milk, which, having been kept ſeveral days, was become very ſour. No complaints were made by the children, nor did any bad effects enſue. Two days afterwards, the mother collected *freſh leaves*, and adminiſtered them in the ſame doſe, as before, and at the ſame hour. At eight o'clock, the children breakfaſted of nettle pottage, that is, oatmeal gruel with freſh nettles boiled in it, a meſs well known in this county. At nine, they began to be uneaſy; were chilly and liſtleſs; yawned much; and frequently ſtretched out their limbs. The oldeſt vomited a little, and complained of gripings in his belly; but the others expreſſed no ſigns of pain. The ſecond child died at ten o'clock; the youngeſt about one; and the oldeſt at three in the afternoon. No agonies accompanied their diſſolution; no ſwelling of the abdomen enſued; and, after death, they had the appearance of being in a placid ſleep. Theſe particulars I learned from the unfortunate parents of the children, whoſe ignorance led them too long, and too fatally to rely on the trifling and inefficacious means of relief, ſuggeſted to them by their neighbours *(b)*.

AN

(b) SEVERAL writers on natural hiſtory have doubted the poiſonous quality of the yew tree; but, in addition to the fact above related, we may adduce the following paſſage from

Cæſar's

AN EXTRA UTERINE FŒTUS VOIDED BY STOOL, TWENTY-TWO YEARS AFTER PREGNANCY.

MRS. —— of Row-Crofs, near Mottram, July 1751, when in the fixth month of her pregnancy, and twenty-fourth year of her age, received a fudden fright, which occafioned a fevere pain in her loins, and was foon fucceeded by a flooding, but without a mifcarriage. Thefe

Cæfar's Commentaries: *Cativulcus, rex dimidiæ partis Eburonum, qui unà cum Ambiorige confilium inierat, ætate jam confectus, quum laborem aut belli aut fugæ ferre non poffet, omnibus precibus, deteftatus Ambiorigem, qui ejus confilii auctorfuiffet,* TAXO, *cujus magna in Galliâ Germaniâque copia eft, fe exanimavit.* Comment. lib. VI. fect. 29.

MR. EVELYN feems to place no dependence on this account, yet he acknowledges, that the yew is *efteemed* noxious to cattle, when it is in the feeds or newly fprouting. "But what is very odd, if true," fays he, "is that which the "late Mr. Aubrey recounts, in his Mifcellanies, of a gentle-"woman that had long been ill, without any benefit from the "phyfician: She dreamed, that a friend of her's, deceafed, "told her mother, that if fhe gave her daughter a drink of "*yew* pounded, fhe fhould recover: It was accordingly "given her, and fhe prefently died. The mother being "almoft diftracted for the lofs of her daughter, her chamber-"maid, to comfort her, faid, *furely, what fhe gave her was* "*not the occafion of her death, and that fhe would adventure on* "*it herfelf:* She did fo, and died!" Evelyn's Silva, Hunter's edition, p. 380.

fymptoms

ſymptoms were relieved by the medicines, then directed for her by an experienced and judicious ſurgeon. But the *abdomen*, afterwards, became much diſtended; and continued ſo about half a year, when it ſubſided all at once, whilſt ſhe was in a recumbent poſture. Her *menſes* in a ſhort time appeared, and returned at the ſtated periods, with ſufficient regularity; but they were always attended with violent pain. Milk alſo flowed from her breaſts during ſeveral years. In 1757, ſhe was afflicted with great flatulence, and often with hyſterical fits, her uterine diſcharges were become very putrid, and her health and ſtrength ſeemed to be gradually impairing. She conſulted me in May 1772; and received great benefit from an emetic, an infuſion of the Peruvian bark, and from frequent doſes of the acid elixir of vitriol. My advice was again deſired in May 1773. At this time, ſhe laboured under the hæmorrhoids; complained of great pain in her loins, and about the *os ſacrum*; had frequent fluſhings in her face; and was much troubled with ſickneſs and thirſt. The apothecary had taken eight ounces of blood from her arm, and had given her ſome aperient medicines. I directed leeches to the hæmorrhoidal veins; an electuary, compoſed of the lenitive electuary and flowers of ſulphur; an infuſion of columbo root; and the following clyſter, to be injected every night at bed-time.

℞. *Ol. è Pedib. Bov.* ℥ *iv. Tinct. Thebaic. V. O. subact.* ʒ *i. M. F. Enema.*

May 12th, SHE began this courſe of medicine.

13th. SHE diſcharged, by the *anus*, two bones of a child's head.

14th. SHE voided, in the ſame way, another bone of the head.

17th. SHE diſcharged the trunk of the body, wanting ſome of the *viſcera* of a female *fœtus*.

19th. SHE parted with a thigh bone. The patient was not, afterwards, ſenſible of any farther diſcharges of this nature.

June 7th. I SAW her: her pains were then abated; her appetite was improved; and her ſtrength ſeemed to be daily increaſing. In this ſtate of convaleſcence, ſhe continued two months; and then, from ſome cauſe which the diſtance of her place of her abode has yet prevented me from learning, ſhe ſuddenly relapſed, and died in a few days.

THE

THE RARITY OF THE AIR A CAUSE OF HÆMORRHAGES.

In the ſecond part of the ſixty-fourth volume of the Philoſophical Tranſactions, Dr. Darwin has favoured the public with ſeveral well conceived experiments, which afford a ſatisfactory proof, that air does not exiſt, in the fluids of the human body, in an elaſtic ſtate; or in ſuch a ſtate as to become elaſtic by any change, yet experienced, in the weight of the incumbent atmoſphere. Hence he concludes, that the accounts of hæmoptöes, and other diſcharges of blood, from perſons who have aſcended high mountains, are either not to be depended upon, or to be aſcribed to violent exerciſe, or to ſome other accidental cauſe.

The relations of ſuch hæmorrhages are too well authenticated, to admit of doubt or controverſy; and they may be explained upon rational and philoſophical principles. The preſſure of the external air muſt be allowed to be a cauſe of reſiſtance to the propulſion of the blood, through the vaſcular ſyſtem. If this preſſure be diminiſhed, and the action of the heart remain the ſame, it is obvious, that the fluids will be propelled with greater force, and that the ſmall veſſels

veſſels will be more diſtended by them. This effect we ſee partially produced by the cupping glaſs, which occaſions a *plethora*, in the veſſels over which it is applied, by diminiſhing the reſiſtance to the circulation of the blood through them. Upon the tops of high mountains, the rarity of the air diminiſhes this reſiſtance univerſally; but thoſe veſſels of the body will be moſt diſtended by the *vis à tergo*, which, belonging to the tendereſt organs, are leaſt capable of reſiſtance. Hence, thoſe of the lungs, noſtrils, eyes, &c. are moſt liable to be ruptured.

HEAT is obſerved to diſtend the veſſels, and to enlarge the bulk of the human body. This effect it produces, not by rarefying the air contained in the blood, but by its expanſile power, and by its ſtimulus on the heart and arteries. All bodies are dilated by heat; and mercury, though freed from air, quicker than almoſt any other.

ELECTRICITY.

WHEN the gout leaves the extremities, and invades other parts of the body, ſinapiſms, bliſters, and volatile epithems are often applied to the wriſts or to the feet, to recal the diſorder to its uſual and natural ſeat. The ſame remedies are

are alſo employed to ſolicit the gout to the extremities, when it has yet made only irregular attacks on the ſyſtem. Might not ſlight, or even ſevere ſhocks of electricity, be highly ſerviceable on ſuch occaſions? The ſtimulating applications, above-mentioned, chiefly affect the ſkin; whereas the electrical ſtroke inſtantly pervades the tendons, articulations, and other internal parts, ſuppoſed to be the ſeat of this diſorder.

In palſies, proceeding from the receſſion of the gout, we ſhould be leſs liable to diſappointment in our expectations from electricity, when thus partially applied, than by the general ſhocks ſo indiſcriminately given.

A POISONOUS SPECIES OF MUSHROOM.

Auguſt 1772. Robert Usherwood, of Middleton, near Mancheſter, a ſtrong healthy man, aged fifty years, early in the morning gathered, and eat what he ſuppoſed to be a muſhroom. He felt no ſymptoms of indiſpoſition till five o'clock in the evening; when, being very thirſty, he drank near a quart of table-beer. Soon afterwards, he became univerſally ſwoln; was ſick; and in great agonies. A ſevere vomitting miting and purging ſucceeded, with violent cramps in his legs and thighs. He diſcharged ſeveral pieces of the *fungus*, but with little or no relief. His pains and evacuations continued, almoſt without intermiſſion, till the next night; when he fell into a ſound ſleep, and awaked, in the morning, perfectly eaſy and free from complaint.

I HAVE ſent to Mr. Hudſon, author of the *Flora Anglica*, a ſpecies of *fungus*, which the poor man thinks exactly reſembles what he ſwallowed. And it appears, to this ingenious botaniſt, to be the *Agaricus Clypeatus* Linn. Spec. Plant. p. 1642, of which there is a good figure in Scheffer's *Icones Fungorum*.

WORMS DISCHARGED FROM THE LUNGS.

MR. JOSEPH HANFORTH, of Stockport, aged forty-nine years, had been long troubled with a cough, and with a fulneſs and oppreſſion at his breaſt. He frequently expectorated lumps of black, grumous blood, which gave him relief. In February 1774, the oppreſſion increaſed, and in the night he diſcharged, by coughing, two maſſes, one of the ſize of a nutmeg, the other ſmaller. They were of the colour of chocolate.

colate. When the larger ſubſtance was opened, it was found to contain a conſiderable number of worms, like maggots, in a very lively ſtate. His cough and expectoration ſtill continue; but the oppreſſion at his breaſt is not ſo troubleſome; and the diſcharge of coagulated blood is leſs frequent. This patient's complaints were not attended with any hectic ſymptoms, and he is unable to give any account of the origin of them. The late Dr. Watſon of Stockport ſaw, and examined the worms which he diſcharged. Schenkius, in his *Obſervationes Medicinales de Pulmonibus*, lib. II. p. 249, relates a caſe ſomewhat ſimilar to that of Mr. Hanforth. The reader may alſo conſult Morgagni, Epiſt. XIX. Art. 41. Epiſt. XXI. Art. 43. *Lieutaud Hiſt. Anat. Med.* vol. II. p. 40, Obſ. 572, p. 79. Obſ. 720.

MILIARY FEVER.

THAT the miliary eruption is *frequently* fabricated by cloſe rooms, heating remedies, and forced ſweats, is a truth acknowledged by almoſt every modern practitioner; and the danger and abſurdity of ſuch a method of treatment, in every ſpecies of fever, cannot be too ſtrongly enforced.

But

But ſome very ingenious phyſicians have ſuppoſed, that the miliary fever, *invariably* and in all *inſtances*, is derived from the cauſes above recited; and they have flattered themſelves and the public, that, by a cooling and antiſeptic regimen, it may be baniſhed entirely from the catalogue of diſeaſes. This is an expectation which, I fear, experience will not warrant. Neither hot rooms, cardiac remedies, nor profuſe ſweating, produce at all times the miliary eruption; and I have ſeen it occur, when the antiphlogiſtic regimen has been purſued to its full extent. Of this the following caſe, which I have ſelected from ſeveral others, affords a ſtriking proof.

February 4th, 1770. Mrs. L. aged 30, laboured under the uſual ſymptoms of a *febricula* or ſlow fever, for which ſhe took ſaline draughts, antimonials, and yeſterday a cathartic, which operated five times. She had four fainting fits previous to this evacuation; and ſoon afterwards a miliary eruption, of the white and red kind, made its appearance on her breaſt, arms, and the trunk of her body. Her pulſe, when I firſt ſaw her, beat a hundred and twenty ſtrokes in a minute, and was extremely feeble; her heat was moderate; her tongue furred; her head painful; and ſhe laboured under a conſtant oppreſſion about the *præcordia*. Her houſe was in an elevated and airy ſituation; the weather was cold;

cold; ſhe lay in a large and well-ventilated chamber, at a diſtance from the fire; and with no more bed clothes than ſhe uſed in health. The following medicine was directed.

℞. *Sp. Mindereri ſeſcunciam; Elix. Paregoric. drachmas tres; Sp. Volat. Aromat. drachmam unam.*

M. Sumantur Cochl. ij. minima, omni ſeſquihora, ex hauſtulo Seri Lactis Vinos. tenuis.

In a few hours, I found her much relieved. She no longer complained of any oppreſſion at her breaſt; her ſkin was moiſt; and her pulſe fuller and ſlower. The miliary eruption was conſiderably increaſed; and her arms and hands were become ſtiff and ſwoln.

It is unneceſſary to proceed with the detail of this caſe, which terminated in the recovery of the patient. The circumſtances related fully evince, that a miliary eruption may occur in a cold ſeaſon of the year; with a free acceſs of air; and under an antiphlogiſtic method of cure.

ANGINA PECTORIS.

In November 1773, I was deſired to viſit a gentleman near Knutsford, in Cheſhire, aged upwards

upwards of fifty; who had been, for ſeveral years, ſubject to frequent attacks of a moſt alarming and oppreſſive ſenſation in his breaſt, which he knew not how to deſcribe. This ſymptom was attended with a pain about the middle of the *ſternum*, inclining to the left ſide; and he was generally affected, at the ſame time, with a pain in his left arm, where the deltoid muſcle is inſerted. As I viſited the patient only once, and took no notes of his caſe, I cannot give a minute detail of it, and muſt content myſelf with ſaying, that I apprehended his diſorder to be what Dr. Heberden hath ſo accurately deſcribed under the name of *Angina Pectoris*. Various anodyne and antiſpaſmodic remedies were preſcribed; but theſe produced only a temporary alleviation of his complaints. And it was obſerved, that nothing afforded ſuch inſtantaneous eaſe, during the paroxyſms of his diſorder, as venæſection or vomiting. In July 1774, he died; and his body was examined by Mr. Allen, an ingenious ſurgeon in Knutsford, who has favoured me with the enſuing account of the diſſection.

The left lobe of the liver was conſiderably enlarged, and full of indurated, white tumors; and nearly one half of the right lobe was beginning to be affected in a ſimilar manner. The gall bladder was diſtended with bile; the ſtomach was

was hard and ſchirrous, as far as it was in contact with the liver; the lungs were pale and livid; and the blood veſſels as diſtinct as if they had been injected with Pruſſian blue. The heart and *aorta deſcendens* were in a ſound ſtate; very little water was found in the pericardium, or mediaſtinum; and there was nothing preternatural in the appearance of the diaphragm.

THIS gentleman had lived freely, but was not ſubject to the gout.

DR. HEBERDEN has favoured me with the following remarks upon this caſe. "The "diſſection of this ſufferer by the *angina pec-* "*toris*, as well as that of a few others, which "I have heard of, teaches us, that the diſeaſe "is neither owing to inflammation, nor to any "mal-conformation of the parts. We muſt "not, therefore, ſeek for the cure amongſt the "means which lower the *vis vitæ*; and we need "not deſpair of finding it elſewhere. But we "ſhould not expect to find it very ſoon, when "we conſider how little ſucceſs has attended all "our ſearches after a remedy for the gout, and "for ſome other diſtempers, with whoſe natures "we have had, for ſome thouſand years, ſuch "abundant means of being acquainted."

A phyſician, in this neighbourhood, informs me, that, a few years ago, he was attacked, about two o'clock in the morning, with a violent oppreſſion in his breathing, accompanied with a pain in the arm, at the inſertion of the *deltoid* muſcle. This complaint recurred, at uncertain intervals, during ſeveral months; and induced him to have an iſſue ſet a little above the knee: But, before this could be ſuppoſed to have afforded any relief, he was ſeized with a bilious *diarrhœa*, which continued near a fortnight, and entirely removed all his complaints; nor has he ever ſince had a return of them. Previouſly to the invaſion of this malady, which ſeems to have had an analogy to the *angina pectoris*, he paſſed ſome time in London, where he lived more luxuriouſly than uſual. Certain ſymptoms of redundancy and acrimony were the conſequences of this mode of life, from which he was perfectly freed by the *diarrhœa*. In this, as in the former caſe, there was no ſuſpicion of gout.

T Y P H U S.

The *typhus* is now prevalent here, and the *eryſipelas* and *cholera morbus* are alſo frequent. I have had many caſes wherein the former has attacked the face and head, in a ſevere degree, in ſtages of the low fever, in which, from the proſtration of ſtrength, ſuch local inflammation could be little expected. Vomitings and purgings,

ings, alſo, have proved very untoward ſymptoms in this diſorder. The latter ſometimes terminate in diſcharges of blood. In the cure of this fever, I have found wine and the dulcified ſpirit of vitriol almoſt univerſally ſalutary. Laudanum, Peruvian bark, bliſters, columbo root, caſcarilla, fixed air, *gummi rubrum aſtringens*, and camphor have proved auxiliaries, I believe, nearly according to the order in which they have been enumerated. The affection of the head is often relieved by opiates, but, in ſome inſtances, is much aggravated by them; and I fear very ſerious miſchief will ariſe from the incautious and indiſcriminate uſe that is now made of them, by theoriſts of a certain medical ſect. The Peruvian bark ſeems to anſwer beſt as a gentle tonic; and, therefore, I uſually adminiſter it in infuſion, rather than in ſubſtance. But, even in this form, the ſtomach is ſometimes offended with it, and accords better with columbo root or caſcarilla. Fixed air is generally grateful to the patient; and, as it covers the taſte of other medicines, interferes not with their action, and probably adds to their efficacy. I often combine the ſalt of tartar with draughts of the infuſion above-mentioned, directing them to be taken, in effervescence, with lemon juice. Camphor I have found a doubtful remedy. If given in a large doſe, it confuſes the head, renders the tongue dry, and creates a diſtreſſing thirſt; and, even in a ſmall doſe, I have ſometimes ſuſpected it of contributing to the production of theſe effects. But, in other inſtances, it has, apparently, been taken with no inconſiderable benefit. The utility of bliſters, in the *typhus* as it now prevails, is confined, I think, to the middle and latter period of the diſorder. The delirium is generally relieved by their application;. and, if the fever be protracted, they ſometimes effect its termination, by inflaming the the ſkin, and diſpoſing it to boils, and other *exanthemata*, which prove a ſort of criſis. I have not mentioned vomits, becauſe the phyſician is ſeldom called early enough to exhibit them, with propriety; for the head quickly becomes ſo exquiſitely tender, as to make every degree of agitation dangerous.

A P O P L E X Y.

In a fit of apoplexy, when the power of ſwallowing ſeems to be loſt, it is ſtill practicable to adminiſter a few grains of tartar emetic, by introducing them, in a dry form, with a tea-ſpoon or *ſpatula*, into the *pharynx*. The medicine will thus paſs, inſenſibly, and without any apparent effort of deglutition, down the gullet into the ſtomach; and,

and, by the action of vomiting, benefit may sometimes be obtained.

SOLUTION OF WATER IN AIR.

An eminent philosopher informed me, some time ago, that the solvent power of air on water, is a discovery of a much older date than is commonly supposed; and that it was well known to Dr. Edmund Halley, about the beginning of the present century. The following quotation which I have extracted from the second volume of Lowthorp's Abridgment of the Philosophical Transactions, will sufficiently evince the truth of this assertion.

"Vapours being raised by warmth, let us, "for a first supposition, put, that the whole "surface of the whole globe were all water very "deep; or, rather, that the whole body of the "earth were water, and that the sun had his "diurnal course about it: I take it, that it would "follow, that the air, of itself, would imbibe a "certain quantity of aqueous vapours, and re-"tain them, *like salts dissolved in water*; that the "sun warming the air, and drawing a more "plentiful vapour from the water, in the day-"time, the air would sustain a greater propor-"tion of vapours, as *warm water will hold more*

" *dissolved salts*, which, upon the absence of the " sun, in the nights, would be all again dis- " charged in dews, *analogous to the precipitation* " *of salts on the cooling of liquors (a).*"

On the 17th of January 1785, though the air was clear and serene, and the sun frequently shone with great brightness, and with a warmth seldom experienced at such a season of the year, yet a very extraordinary degree of moisture manifested itself in the foot-paths, streets, and on the walls of buildings. In the vestibule of my dwelling-house, the flags were as wet as if they had been washed, small lakes of water lodged upon the oil cloths across the floor, and streams trickled down the walls, which, being well painted, were incapable of absorption. But the wainscot doors and the architraves surrounding them were much less affected by the moisture. From what cause proceeded this superabundant deposition of aqueous vapour? From the same cause, I apprehend, which, in summer, covers with moisture a glass decanter or silver tankard filled with any liquor. The air was saturated with water, conveyed into these regions by

(a) See Lowthorp's Abridg. of Phil. Transf. vol. II. p. 127.

a warm

a warm ſouth wind, after a very long continued and ſevere froſt; and was clear and ſerene, becauſe this water was perfectly diſſolved. But flags, ſtone, and brick long retain their temperature; and, in their gradual acquiſition of warmth from the atmoſphere, they muſt diminiſh the menſtrual power of ſuch portions of air, as come ſucceſſively into contact with them. Hence, the air will diſcharge upon them what it held before in *chemical ſolution*. And, as this may greatly exceed, in quantity, what ſubſiſts, at any time, in a ſtate of *diffuſion*, much more moiſture will manifeſt itſelf, under the circumſtances above deſcribed, than even in a miſty ſtate of the atmoſphere.

When a ſouth wind blows immediately after a ſharp froſt, a white efflореſcence is often obſervable on the outſide walls of houſes, &c. This ariſes from a ſimilar depoſition of atmoſpheric moiſture, converted into a hoar froſt, by the cold of the buildings on which it is received. The wainſcot doors and architraves, though painted, were leſs affected with moiſture than the walls. For wood, being a very ſlow conductor of heat, muſt be leſs capable of diminiſhing the diſſolvent power of the air; and, conſequently, occaſion little or no precipitation from it.

That the air is capable of containing immenſe quantities of water, with perfect tranſparency, is evident from the preceding obſervations. The Biſhop of Landaff, who has alſo aſcertained this fact from other *data*, calculates, that, were the whole precipitated which is diſſolved in the atmoſphere, it might probably be ſufficient to cover the earth, to the depth of above thirty feet. So that we may very juſtly be ſaid, even in the faireſt weather, to walk in an ocean.

In November of the preceding year, I noticed a great, and almoſt inſtantaneous alteration in the temperature of the atmoſphere, by a ſudden change of the wind from north to ſouth, after having continued many days in the former direction. At the time of this occurrence, I was on a journey: The ſun ſhone bright, and the air was clear: But when I firſt perceived the ſenſation of chillineſs, a ſlight miſt appeared, which, however, ſoon diffuſed itſelf and became inviſible. Yet the cold increaſed progreſſively, as far as I could judge from feeling, without the aid of a thermometer. May not this cold be aſcribed to the ſolution of the aqueous vapours, brought, by the ſoutherly wind, into air diveſted of its uſual proportion of water, in the regions of the north, from which it flowed? It is related in the Memoirs of the Royal Academy of Sciences for 1709, that the cold, which ſunk the mercury to the

the fifth degree of Fahrenheit's ſcale, on the 13th of January, came on at Paris, with a gentle wind from the ſouth; and that it was diminiſhed when the wind increaſed and turned to the north. M. de la Hire advances, as the ſolution of this phænomenon, that the mountains of Auvergne, which are to the ſouth of Paris, were, at that time, covered with ſnow. But M. Homberg accounts for it, by obſerving, that the ſouth wind was only a reflux of the ſame cold air, which had been previouſly blown from the north *(a)*. It is ſurely very unphiloſophical to ſuppoſe, that the ſame air in its regreſs from a ſouthern, ſhould be colder than in its progreſs from a northern latitude. And, in the fact which I have related, to which other analogous ones might be added, no ſnow ſubſiſted to occaſion the change of temperature *(b)*. Whoever goes into a room or paſſes through a ſtreet, in the ſummer ſeaſon, which has juſt been waſhed, will perceive effects exactly ſimilar; and can be at no loſs for a rational explanation of them.

(a) See Templeman's Abridgment of the Memoirs of the Academy of Sciences, vol. II. p. 244.

(b) See Philoſophical Tranſ. vol. LXI. p. 216.

AFFEC-

AFFECTIONS OF THE EYES.

MR. WARD, aged forty-eight years, formerly an attorney, and a very ſtudious man, has been gradually loſing his eye-ſight during twenty years; and is now capable only of diſtinguiſhing light from darkneſs. The pupils of his eyes are more dilated than is natural, in the dark; and they are contracted, in an equal proportion, in a ſtrong light. There is a ſmall ſpeck or obſcurity juſt diſcernible in the centre of the pupil of the left eye, like an incipient cataract, but inſufficient to affect viſion in a material degree. He has ſuffered no pain in his eyes, and can aſcribe his blindneſs to no other cauſe, but cloſe ſtudy and application. Can this diſeaſe be denominated a *gutta ſerena?* It ſeems to be ſeated in the *retina*; but, from the ready contraction, and dilatation of the pupils, it ſhould appear, that the nerves are ſtrongly affected by the *ſtimulus* of light, and yet are incapable of conveying to the mind the uſual ſenſations produced by luminous objects. In palſies, ſuch partial affections of the nerves ſometimes occur.

THE Rev. Mr. S. of Rochdale informs me, that the pupils of his eyes do not ſenſibly contract in the light, or dilate in the dark. And he he obſerves, that much more light is requiſite to him, for diſtinct viſion, than to others, whoſe eyes are differently formed. In the duſk of the evening, when others ſee tolerably well, he can ſcarcely diſtinguiſh any objects. The pupils of his eyes are very ſmall.

ASYLUM OR LOCK HOSPITAL.

An Aſylum, or Lock Hoſpital, for the reception of female patients labouring under the venereal diſeaſe, has been lately eſtabliſhed at Mancheſter; and it is to be wiſhed, that ſo laudable an example may be followed in other places. To ſhew the utility of ſuch inſtitutions, and to obviate the objections which have been made to them, the following advertiſements were written, and are prefixed to the two REPORTS of the hoſpital above-mentioned.

MANCHESTER, 1774.

Whoever reflects on the variety of diſeaſes to which the human body is incident, will find, with concern, that a conſiderable part of them is derived from immoderate paſſions and vicious indulgences. Sloth, intemperance, and irregular

irregular defires are the great fources of evil, which contract the duration, and imbitter the enjoyment of life. But humanity, whilft fhe mourns over the vices of mankind, incites us to alleviate the miferies which flow from them. The private hand of charity is never fhut, when ficknefs, complicated with poverty, prefents itfelf; and hofpitals are eftablifhed, in every part of the kingdom, for the reception of the wretched, whether innocent or guilty.

A NEW inftitution, founded on thefe benevolent principles, confonant to found policy, and favourable to the interefts of virtue, now claims the attention, and encouragement of the public: The object of it is to provide relief for a loathfome and painful diftemper, often fatal when neglected, but which admits of an almoft certain cure, when the patient is under confinement, and fubject to proper regulations. This afylum, it may reafonably be hoped, will withdraw from their haunts thofe wretches, who feduce unwary youth, contaminate them with difeafe, fpread wide infection, and entail fhame and mifery on a feeble pofterity. To the penitent fufferers it will afford a pleafing refuge, will give opportunity to confirm their wavering refolutions, and will reftore them to health, to peace, and ufefulnefs. Happy will the governors be in difmiffing fuch with this benevolent injunction:

GO, AND SIN NO MORE.

1775.

THE

PREFACE.

THE three preceding parts of this work comprehend the whole of what is inſerted in the author's former volumes of Medical, Philoſophical, and Experimental Eſſays. To the preſent edition he has thought it expedient, to annex various miſcellaneous communications, which have been publiſhed in the Tranſactions of the Royal Society, and of the College of Phyſicians; in the Memoirs of the Mancheſter Literary Society, and in thoſe of the Medical Society of London; in the London Medical

Journal; in the Medical Commentaries of Edinburgh; in the two Annual Registers; and in the Gentleman's Magazine. The arrangement, with a few exceptions, is regulated according to the order here laid down; and a few pieces are inserted, which have not before been offered to the public.

MANCHESTER, JUNE 12, 1789.

ESSAY I.

ON A

NEW AND CHEAP METHOD OF

PREPARING POT-ASH,

WITH REMARKS.

Addressed to the Earl *of* Stamford, *President of the* Agricultural Society *at* Manchester *(a)*.

THE Agricultural Society at Manchester, has long recommended the making of reservoirs, for the water which flows from dunghills, in farm-yards. This water is strongly impregnated with the salts and putrid matter of the dunghill; and, by stagnation, acquires a much higher degree of putrescency, and probably becomes proportionably more replete with salts. When thus collected and improved, it is pumped

(a) Inserted in the Philosoph. Transf. vol. LXX. p. 545; and in the Annual Register, for 1780, p. 120.

into

into an hogſhead, which, being drawn upon a ſledge or ſmall cart, is conveyed into the meadows, for the purpoſe of ſprinkling them with this rich manure. This important improvement in rural œconomy, I apprehend, has not been extended much beyond the diſtrict of our Society; and it ſeems to be unknown to one of the lateſt, and moſt intelligent writers on huſbandry. For Lord Kaims, in a recent work on this ſubject, of which he has favoured me with a copy, has not even mentioned it.

But theſe reſervoirs may be applied to a purpoſe ſtill more ſubſervient to public utility, than that above deſcribed. Joſiah Birch, Eſq. a gentleman who carries on an extenſive manufactory, and bleaches his own yarn, about ſix months ago, was induced, by a happy turn of thought, to try whether the dunghill water might not be converted into pot-aſhes. He accordingly evaporated a large quantity of it, and burnt the *reſiduum* in an oven; the product of which ſo perfectly anſwered his expectations, that he has ever ſince continued to prepare theſe aſhes, and to employ them in the proceſs of bucking. A ſtranger to that narrowneſs of ſpirit, which ſeeks the concealment of a lucrative diſcovery, he is deſirous that it ſhould be communicated both to this and to the Royal Society; and has furniſhed

me

me with the following account, together with the plan annexed (*b*).

"The quantity of muck water uſed, was "twenty-four wine pipes full; which employed

(*b*)

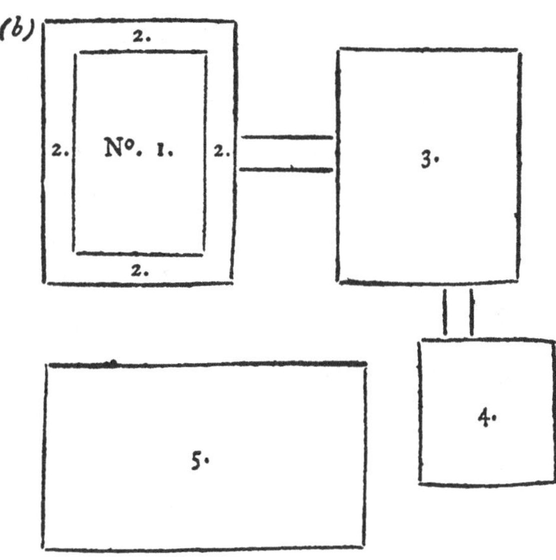

" N°. 1. The dunghill.

" 2. A ſough or drain, round the bottom of the dunghill.

" 3. A hole, or pit, to receive the muck water from N°. 1.

" 4. A well, to receive the muck water from the pit, " wherein a pump is fixed to convey it to the pan, N°. 5, " in which it is boiled to the conſiſtence of treacle, and after- " wards burned in an oven. The pan, N°. 5, is formed at " the bottom of iron plates; and turned up a little round the " edges, to which deal planks are ſcrewed, ſo as to make " it about twenty inches in depth."

 "a man

"a man and two horſes two days, to cart it "from the pump to the pan wherein it was "boiled: but this expence I ſhall now ſave, "as I ſhall lay a ſough of brick, which will con- "vey it from the ſough to the boiler. The "coals, uſed to boil and burn it, were one hun- "dred and twenty baſkets; and I ſuppoſe each "baſket weighs ſix ſcore pounds, or upwards. "One man was occupied, three weeks, in boiling "and burning. The quantity of aſhes made "was 9 cwt. 1 qr. 12 lb. well worth, at the "preſent price of aſhes here, two guineas per "hundred.

"9 cwt. 1 qr. 12 lb. at 42 s. per cwt. -		£19 : 13 : 0
"A man and two horſes, two days, at 6 s. - - -	£0 : 12 : 0	
"120 baſkets of coals, at 5 d. per baſket, - -	2 : 10 : 0	
"A man's wages for three weeks	1 : 7 : 0	
		£ 4 : 9 : 0
		£15 : 4 : 0

"The gain therefore amounts to £15 : 4 : 0, "deducting only a trifle for the wear of the pan "and oven."

The profits ariſing from this preparation of pot-aſh, are ſufficiently evinced by the foregoing eſtimate; and they may, perhaps, admit of increaſe by future improvements. In the ſpring and ſummer ſeaſons, I ſhould ſuppoſe, the evaporation

poration might be carried on, without the aid of fire; by conveying the dunghill water from the reſervoir, through proper ſluices, into ſhallow troughs or ponds, of ſuch extent as to afford a ſufficient ſurface for the action of the ſun and wind. Theſe might be covered, in rainy weather, with awnings of canvaſs, painted on the outſide black, and white on the inſide; the former with a view to abſorb, the latter to reflect the rays of light.

THIS pot-aſh is of a greyiſh white appearance, deliqueſces a little in moiſt air, but if kept in a dry room near the fire, acquires a powdery ſurface. It is hard, and of a ſpongy texture when broken, with many ſmall cryſtals in its ſubſtance. The colour of its internal parts is duſky, and variegated. To the taſte, it is acrid, ſaline, and ſulphureous. It emits no ſmell of volatile alkali either in a ſolid form, diſſolved, or when added to lime water; neither does it communicate the ſapphire colour to a ſolution of blue vitriol. Silver is quickly tinged black by it, a proof that it contains much phlogiſton. Ten grains of this pot-aſh required eleven drops of the weak ſpirit of vitriol to ſaturate them: The like quantity of ſalt of tartar required, of the ſame acid, twenty-four drops. A ſtrong efferveſcence occurred in both mixtures: From the former, a ſulphureous vapour was exhaled. A tea-ſpoonful of the ſyrup of violets, diluted with an ounce of water, was changed into a bright green colour by five grains of the ſalt of tartar; but ten grains of this new pot-aſh were neceſſary to produce the ſame hue in a ſimilar mixture. Half an ounce of the pot-aſh diſſolved entirely in half a pint of hot water; but, when the liquor was cold, a large purple ſediment ſubſided to the bottom: And it was found, that this ſediment amounted to about two thirds of the whole quantity of aſhes uſed.

I HAVE not leiſure, at preſent, to proſecute theſe experiments farther; and ſhall, therefore, content myſelf with making a few general obſervations on the facts which have been advanced.

1. THIS pot-aſh is a true fixed vegetable alkali, and a product of putrefaction which has not, that I recollect, been noticed by the chemiſts. A very celebrated writer has even aſſerted, in expreſs terms, that "all vegetables, not "excepting thoſe which in their natural ſtate "furniſh aſhes containing much fixed alkali, "when burnt, after their acid has been altered "by a complete putrefaction, leave aſhes en"tirely free from alkali *(c)*."

2. THE quantity of alkali contained in this pot-aſh may, with ſome probability, be eſtimated at about one-third of its weight; whereas the

(c) Macquer's Dictionary of Chemiſtry, Article ALKALI.

white

white Mufcovy afhes are faid to yield only one-eighth part *(d)*. Of its impurities, fulphur is the moft injurious to its bleaching powers; and fhould, in the preparation of it, be carefully feparated. A longer-continued, and more gentle calcination, in a furnace fupplied with a fufficient current of air, might, perhaps, anfwer this end. But the moft effectual method would be to lixiviate the falts with pure water, after a moderate fufion, and then to evaporate them flowly to drynefs. It muft however be remarked, that, in thus freeing the pot-afh from phlogiftic matter, another impurity is generated. For both the action of fire, and the folution in water, convert, into earth, a portion of the alkaline falt.

3. No quick-lime appears to be contained in this pot-afh; for a folution of it, poured from its fediment, remained clear, though long expofed to the air. Nor did it acquire any milkinefs by being blown into from the lungs. But perhaps the addition of this cauftic fubftance, in a due proportion, would increafe its activity and value, when employed in many of the arts. For the Ruffian pot-afh is more pungent to the tafte, faturates a larger proportion of acid, and diffolves oils more powerfully than the purer

(d) Home on Bleaching, p. 157.

alkaline ſalts. And Dr. Home has proved *(e)*, that theſe qualities depend on a large admixture of quick-lime.

4. It would be worthy of trial to aſcertain, whether the large purple ſediment, which ſubſides when this pot-aſh is lixiviated, might not be applied to the manufacture of Pruſſian blue; or uſed, in the manner recommended by Mr. Macquer, for dying wool and ſilk. See the Memoirs of the French Academy for the year 1749 *(f)*.

5. The farmer, though he live at a diſtance from the manufactures in which pot-aſh is employed, may find his account in preparing it from dunghill water. For it will furniſh him with a top-dreſſing, for his garden and land, of great fertilizing powers. But if fuel be dear where he reſides, and neceſſaries wanting for the conſtruction of a furnace, the ſimple evaporation of the water may ſuffice. And the putrid lye, thus reduced to a ſolid form, will prove to be a rich manure. At Hart-Hill, my ſummer abode, about three miles from Mancheſter, I have lately practiſed a method of making a compoſt of dunghill water. The weeds and rakings of the garden, the dreſſings of the fields, the leaves

(e) Eſſay on Bleaching.

(f) See alſo Neumann's Chemiſtry, by Lewis.

blown

blown from the trees, and other refuſe matters, are put together near the reſervoir; out of which the water is occaſionally pumped, and ſcattered over the heap. So ſtrong a ferment almoſt inſtantly excites putrefaction; and theſe vegetable ſubſtances are ſoon converted into a fertile mould, which, retaining the ſalts and oils of the dunghill water, ſuffers the ſuperfluous moiſture to exhale into the air, or to percolate through it. And I have found by experience, that the compoſt, thus prepared, is laid on the meadows at leſs expence, and that it is more efficacious and durable in its operation, than the ſprinklings which, at ſtated times, they formerly received. For my land, though good, and in fine condition, is light and ſandy; and the dunghill water quickly paſſed below the roots of the vegetables, which grow upon its ſurface.

POSTSCRIPT.

IT has been ſuggeſted to me, that the foregoing diſcovery has no claim to the patronage of the Agricultural Society, becauſe, in this manufacturing county, it may, eventually, tend to check the cultivation of land, by robbing it of one ſpecies of manure. But I conceive the operation of it will be entirely the reverſe: For it will promote the collection of every putrescent article, and thus augment the farmer's dunghill, at the same time that it excites a more universal attention to the preservation of muck water; the reservoirs for which are yet few, and have been made chiefly by those who follow husbandry for amusement, and not as an occupation. The public therefore will be gainers both by the saving, and by the acquisition; and a two-fold branch of rural œconomy will be established, at once lucrative to the husbandman, and important to the artist and manufacturer.

BUT, admitting all the supposed force of the allegation, it must surely be acknowledged, that the main design of our institution is to increase the productiveness of agriculture, by stimulating the farmer to every beneficial undertaking, consistent with his profession. Now in this case, the *beneficial* is best measured by the Hudibrastic standard: For,

"What's the value of a thing,
"But so much money as 'twill bring?"

I TRUST, therefore, that the Society will not, by declining to patronize the present discovery, justify the sarcasm of an ingenious poet of this place, who has humorously charged some of us with teaching,

"By crops increas'd, and profits less,
"The way t' enrich the nation."

ESSAY

ESSAY II.

ON THE

FATAL EFFECTS

OF

PICKLES

INPREGNATED WITH COPPER *(a)*.

NOTWITHSTANDING the repeated warnings, that have been offered to the public, concerning thoſe inſidious poiſons, which gain an eaſy, becauſe an unſuſpected, admiſſion into the human body *(b)*, few precautions have hitherto been taken againſt their baneful effects.

(a) Communicated to Sir George Baker, Bart. and inſerted in the Medical Tranſactions of the College of Phyſicians, vol. III. p. 80.

(b) See Sir George Baker's valuable papers in the Medical Tranſactions; Dr. Falconer's Obſervations on Copper; and the Experiments and Obſervations on the Poiſon of Lead, in vol. I.

Copper

Copper and lead, in one form or other, are employed in the conſtruction of almoſt every culinary utenſil; and, as theſe metals have been fully proved to be injurious to our ſyſtem, the careleſs uſe of them puts us in daily hazard, not only of the loſs of health, but even of life itſelf. A melancholy inſtance, of this kind, has lately fallen under my obſervation; and I ſhall briefly relate the particulars of it, as the caſe is not only curious and affecting, but furniſhes a ſalutary admonition to mankind.

On Monday, Auguſt 25, 1783, a young lady, ſeventeen years of age, amuſed herſelf, whilſt under the hands of the hair-dreſſer, with eating pickled ſamphire; of which ſhe conſumed two breakfaſt-plates full, amounting to three or four ounces. Being very thirſty, ſoon afterwards, ſhe drank about the fifth part of a pint of vinegar. In the evening, ſhe complained of pain in her ſtomach, and perceived a raſh upon her hands and breaſt. She went to bed early, felt indiſpoſed, and ſlept little during the night. The raſh almoſt entirely diſappeared before Tueſday noon. She was troubled, at times, with ſhooting pains over her whole body, but particularly on the right ſide; and was dejected, reſtleſs, and very thirſty. On Wedneſday, the pain and thirſt continued, ſhe expreſſed a longing for acids, and was much troubled with flatulence.

flatulence. Her pulſe was frequent and ſmall, her tongue covered with a white fur, and ſhe paſſed ſeveral days without a ſtool. During the operation of a laxative mixture, the pain removed from the right ſide to the left, and ſhe felt a great and univerſal ſoreneſs. On Thurſday, the ſymptoms continued without abatement. The ſucceeding day, the pain in her ſide became extremely violent; in the evening, however, it was alleviated, and never afterwards returned with much ſeverity. On Saturday morning, ſickneſs came on; ſhe vomited, at intervals, through the day; and a hiccup uſually preceded her retchings. The matters diſcharged were not offenſive, and conſiſted chiefly of the liquids ſhe ſwallowed. The retchings were inceſſant on Sunday morning; a quantity of ſamphire was thrown up; and the diſcharges were of a green colour, very offenſive, and taſted like copper to the patient. The hiccup was frequent, and always occaſioned vomiting.

Such had been the progreſſive effects of the poiſon, ſwallowed by this young lady, according to the information of her intelligent apothecary *(c)*; when I was called to her aſſiſtance, in conſultation with an ingenious phyſician of this town *(d)*. She had neglected to ſolicit any

(c) Mr. Bill. *(d)* Dr. Mitchell.

medical

medical aid, till Wednefday; and, then, imprudently concealed the caufe of her complaints. Remedies, however, well adapted to the apparent indications of the cafe, had been affiduoufly adminiftered; and fome of them feemed to afford confiderable relief. When I firft faw her, the difcharges, by ftool and vomiting, were extremely offenfive. The latter were of a dufky green colour, and acid to the patient's tafte, though not perceptibly fo to the noftrils of the by-ftanders. The ftomach was enormoufly diftended with wind, and exquifitely tender to the touch; the hiccupings were almoft inceffant; and the pulfe was quick, tremulous, and irregular. Small dofes of calcined magnefia were given, at proper intervals, in a pleafant emulfion of poppy feeds, with a few drops of laudanum. A truce to the vomiting, pains, hiccup, and other fymptoms fucceeded. But the remiffion was fallacious. In twenty-four hours, the vomiting recurred, with great inquietude; the extremities became cold; the pulfe weak and fluttering; the countenance ghaftly; and fhe expired early on Wednefday morning, September the third. Her body was opened, the fame day, by Mr. Bill; and I was prefent, together with my fon, at the diffection. We found about a quart of brown, fetid liquor in the ftomach. The internal coat of that organ was inflamed and gangrenous, particularly

particularly about the *cardia* and *pylorus*; and this appearance extended itſelf ſome way down the *duodenum*. The liver was ſound; and it was not thought neceſſary to proſecute the examination any farther.

As the pickled ſamphire was freſh, without any thing peculiar in its flavour; and had been eaten, with impunity, by the family in which the young lady reſided, I was, at firſt, inclined to ſuppoſe, that the injury done by it might ariſe, principally, from its quantity as a ſolid acid, and the conſequent degree of irritation on the coats of the ſtomach. But, though this, probably, contributed to its deleterious effects, I found afterwards, by the uſual chemical teſts, that the pickle was very ſtrongly impregnated with copper: And to this cauſe the fatal cataſtrophe muſt chiefly be aſcribed *(e)*.

THE progreſs of the ſymptoms, in the caſe which I have related, is conſonant to the well known action of the poiſon of copper on the human body. A few years ago, I was a witneſs to ſimilar ſufferings, experienced by a braſs foun-

(e) THE volatile alkali is uſually employed to aſcertain the preſence of copper; but, as a teſt, it is much inferior to a piece of poliſhed iron (ſuch as the blade of a knife, &c.) immerſed in the ſuſpected liquor. For there are ſeveral preparations of copper, which exhibit no *blue* colour, on the addition of the volatile ſpirit of ſal ammoniac; but, I believe, no one is known, that will not give a cupreous cruſt to poliſhed iron.

 der

der in Manchefter, a healthy and robuft young man, who was affected with immoderate thirft, violent pain, diftenfion of the ftomach, and fevere retchings, occafioned by drinking water out of an old tea-kettle, the infide of which was covered with verdigrife. I examined the kettle, and obferved a green cruft fpread over its whole internal furface. This man was relieved by caftor oil. A boy, who fwallowed a halfpenny, was fo fick, the fucceeding day, that he could retain nothing upon his ftomach. He vomited a large quantity of a green coloured fluid, which had the fmell of verdigrife. His ficknefs ceafed, he was directed to eat heartily of folid food, and to ufe violent exercife during the courfe of the day. In the evening a clyfter was injected; and, with the ftool that followed it, the halfpenny was difcharged.

The internal ufe of blue vitriol, in no inconfiderable dofes, has been lately recommended by fome bold practitioners. Though I am not an enemy to the cautious ufe of very active remedies, I cannot but entertain apprehenfions, that this promifes no benefits adequate to the danger which it may occafion. The moft dreadful convulfions, I ever beheld, were produced by this preparation of copper, in a young woman, who fwallowed about two drachms of it in a fit of defperation. By the exhibition of evacuants, demulcents, and of fuch abforbents, as have the power of decompofing metallic falts, fhe happily recovered.

recovered. In the interval of her fits, ſhe was perfectly rational. And this caſe, with that of the young lady, firſt recited, and others I could mention, in which arſenick had been taken, ſeems to evince, that it is the common property of mineral poiſons, and not peculiar to that of lead, to exert their baneful operations on the nervous ſyſtem, without injuring the underſtanding or occaſioning delirium, till the patient becomes ſo affected, as in other diſtempers, by the near approach of death.

THE eruption, that appeared in conſequence of the irritation of the ſamphire, is a common ſymptom of acrimony in the ſtomach; and furniſhes both a diagnoſtic, and an indication of cure, which a ſagacious phyſician will not overlook. If aſſiſtance had been called in this early ſtage of the young lady's diſorder, an emetic might, probably, have obviated its fatal termination. But, when the action of any poiſon has been protracted, and the efforts of nature to free herſelf from it, though at firſt ſalutary, are become immoderate, it will be expedient to check the retchings, to allay the pain, and to compoſe the general perturbation of the ſyſtem. A few years ago, a gentleman of rank in this county, chewed and ſwallowed about twenty of the ſeeds of the *ricinoides*, or caſtor nut of Barbadoes. Very violent evacuations, both upwards and downwards, enſued. An emetic was adminiſtered under theſe circumſtances, which aggravated all the ſymptoms. Opium, muſk, and other cordials, were afterwards given without effect. The patient's ſtrength was exhauſted; various ſpaſmodic affections came on; and he died in great agonies. If the injury have been done by any metallic ſalt, which hath an acid for its baſis, calcined magneſia will decompoſe it; and, at the ſame time, gently contribute to carry downwards the offending matter. This preparation, alſo, abates flatulence, corrects the putrefaction of the bile, and thus, in ſeveral ways, may prove an antidote to the operation of different mineral poiſons. Dr. Akenſide has recorded the hiſtory of a woman, who ſwallowed a drachm of corroſive ſublimate yet happily recovered under his judicious treatment. *Idoneis intervallis*, ſays he, *præcepi, in juſculum ovinum ut copioſe inſtillaretur lixivium tartari, atque ita frequentèr epotaretur: Fore enim ſperavi, ut ſal illud alcalinum, cum mercurio corroſivo, in inteſtinis, commiſtum, ſalia ejus acida ad ſe arriperet, & mercurium crudum ferè & innocuum redderet: Quod ex ſententia ſucceſſit. Poſtquam enim, per duodecim dies, in hoc regimine perſtitiſſet, ab omni periculo & dolore liberata eſt (b).*

The *lixivium tartari* was well adapted, according to the laws of chemical affinity, to produce

(b) Akenſide de Dyſenteria, p. 44.

the

the effect, which the excellent physician, who prescribed it, had in view. But it has an offensive taste, and possesses a considerable degree of acrimony; and, on these accounts, is a much less eligible remedy than calcined magnesia, at a time when the patient is so disposed to nausea, and when the stomach and bowels are in a state of the most exquisite sensibility. In such cases, mutton suet is preferable, as a demulcent, to oil; because it is more inviscating, and may be taken in large quantities, without disgust to the palate, when dissolved in barley water. But, if arsenic be the poison to be counteracted, it may be administered in milk, which is said to be a powerful solvent of that mineral *(i)*. To avoid rancidity, a very gentle heat should be employed in melting the suet; and, if the operation be performed in a brass pan, care should be taken that it is lined with pure tin; or covered with the lately invented enamel of fusible spar and gypsum *(k)*.

All fat substances are peculiarly disposed to acquire a cupreous impregnation; and it is much to be lamented, that so little attention is paid, in domestic œconomy, to this well known fact. I suffered very severe sickness, not long since,

(i) See a Treatise of M. P. Toussant Navier, Physician to the King of France.

(k) See London Medical Journal, vol. II. p. 411.

from eating the white ſauce of a calf's head haſh, which I ſuſpected to have received a taint of this nature; and, if ſufficient precautions be not uſed in private families, concerning this point, may we not ſuppoſe, that the evil is much greater in ſhips, hoſpitals, and pariſh work-houſes? An ingenious writer has advanced many arguments to ſhew, that the uſe of copper veſſels in the navy, is one principal cauſe of the ſea ſcurvy *(l)*. And, though I am not inclined to adopt his concluſions in their full extent, yet I think it cannot be denied, that the quantity of verdigriſe, which he has ſhewn to be ſo frequently mixed with the mariner's beef and pork, may produce a prediſpoſition to that diſeaſe, by its action on the nervous ſyſtem, and, particularly, by the injury it does to the powers of digeſtion. It is to be wiſhed, therefore, that iron pans were ſubſtituted for thoſe of copper, both in his majeſty's navy, and in the ſhips of merchants. They are cheaper, more durable, leſs ſubject to foulneſs, and yield nothing from their ſurface, that would prove inſalubrious. And the ſame improvement might be extended, with much advantage, to hoſpitals, work-houſes, and even to private families.

MANCHESTER, SEPTEMBER 25, 1783.

(l) London Medical Obſervations, vol. II. p. 1.

ESSAY

ESSAY III.

SPECULATIONS ON THE PERCEPTIVE POWER OF VEGETABLES (a).

- - - - Theſe are not idle philoſophic dreams;
Full Nature *teems* with life. - - - -

THOMSON's Spring, ſecond edit. line 136 *.

IN all our inquiries into truth, whether natural or moral, it is neceſſary to take into previous conſideration, the kind of evidence which the ſubject admits of; and the degree of it, which is ſufficient to afford ſatisfaction to the mind. Demonſtrative evidence is abſolute, and without

(a) INSERTED in the Memoirs of the Literary and Philoſophical Society of Mancheſter, vol. II. p. 114.

* THESE lines are omitted in the ſubſequent editions of Thomſon's Seaſons.

gradation; but probable evidence aſcends, by regular ſteps, from the loweſt preſumption, to the higheſt moral certainty. A ſingle preſumption is, indeed, of little weight; but a ſeries of ſuch imperfect proofs may produce the fulleſt conviction. The ſtrength of belief, however, may often be greater than is proportionate to the force and number of theſe proofs, either individually or collectively conſidered. For, as uncertainty is always painful to the underſtanding, very ſlight evidence, if the ſubject be capable of no other, ſometimes amounts to credibility. This every philoſopher experiences, in his reſearches into nature; and the obſervation may ſerve as an apology for the following *jeu d'eſprit*; in which I ſhall attempt to ſhew, by the ſeveral analogies of organization and life; inſtinct; ſpontaneity; and ſelf-motion, that plants, like animals, are endued with the powers, both of perception and enjoyment.

I. VEGETABLES bear ſo near a ſimilitude to animals in their STRUCTURE, that botaniſts have derived from anatomy and phyſiology, almoſt all the terms employed in the deſcription of them. A tree or ſhrub, they inform us, conſiſts of a cuticle, cutis, and cellular membrane; of veſſels variouſly diſpoſed, and adapted to the tranſmiſſion of different fluids; and of a ligneous, or bony ſubſtance, covering and defending ſending a pith or marrow. Such organization evidently belongs not to inanimate matter; and when we obſerve, in vegetables, that it is connected with, or inſtrumental to the powers of growth, of ſelf-preſervation, of motion, and of ſeminal increaſe, we cannot heſitate to aſcribe to them a LIVING PRINCIPLE. And by admitting this attribute, we advance a ſtep higher in the analogy we are purſuing. For, the idea of life naturally implies ſome degree of perceptivity: And wherever perception reſides, a greater or leſs capacity for enjoyment ſeems to be its neceſſary adjunct. Indefinite and low, therefore, as this capacity may be, in each ſingle herb or tree, yet, when we conſider the amazing extent of the vegetable kingdom, "from the cedar of Lebanon to the hyſſop upon the wall," the aggregate of happineſs, produced by it, will be found to exceed our moſt enlarged conceptions. It is prejudice only, which reſtrains or ſuppreſſes the delightful emotions, reſulting from the belief of ſuch a diffuſion of good. And, becauſe the framers of ſyſtems have invented arrangements and diviſions of the works of God, to aid the mind in the purſuits of ſcience, we implicitly admit as reality, what is merely artificial; and adopt diſtinctions, without proof of any eſſential difference. *Lapides creſcunt; vegetabilia creſcunt et vivunt; animalia creſcunt, vivunt, et ſentiunt.* This climax, of Linnæus,

Linnæus, is conformable to the doctrines of Ariſtotle, Pliny, Jungius, and others: But none of theſe great men have adduced ſufficient evidence, to ſupport the negative characteriſtics, if I may ſo expreſs myſelf, on which the three kingdoms of nature are here eſtabliſhed. That a gradation ſubſiſts, in the ſcale of beings, is clearly manifeſt; but the higher advances we make in phyſical knowledge, the nearer will the degrees be ſeen to approach each other. And it is no very extravagant conjecture to ſuppoſe, that, in ſome future period, perceptivity may be diſcovered to extend, even beyond the limits now aſſigned to vegetable life. Corallines, madrepores, millepores, and ſpunges were formerly conſidered as foſſil bodies: But the experiments of Count Marſigli evinced, that they are endued with life, and led him to claſs them with the maritime plants. And the obſervations of Ellis, Juſſieu and Peyſonel, have ſince raiſed them to the rank of animals *(b)*. The detection of error, in long eſtabliſhed opinions concerning one branch of natural knowledge, juſtifies the ſuſpicion of its exiſtence in others, which are

(b) CONSULT the Philoſ. Tranſ. Amœnitat. Acad. and particularly the admirable Treatiſe, of Biſhop Watſon, on the SUBJECTS OF CHEMISTRY, printed, but not publiſhed, in 1771; and now inſerted, with additions, in the fifth volume of his Chemical Eſſays, p. 103.

nearly

nearly allied to it: And it will appear, from the proſecution of our inquiry into the inſtincts, ſpontaneity, and ſelf-moving power of vegetables, that the ſuſpicion is not without foundation.

II. INSTINCT is a propenſity, or movement to ſeek, without deliberation, what is agreeable to the particular nature, actuated by it; and to avoid what is incongruous, or hurtful. It is a practical power, which requires no previous knowledge or experience; and which purſues a preſent or future good, without any definite ideas or foreſight; and, often, with very faint degrees of conſciouſneſs. The calf, when it firſt comes into the world, applies to the teats of the cow, utterly ignorant of the taſte, or nutritious quality of the milk, and conſequently, with no views, either to ſenſual gratification, or ſupport: and the duckling, which has been hatched under a hen, at a diſtance from water, diſcovers a conſtant reſtleſſneſs and impatience; and is obſerved to practiſe all the motions of ſwimming, though a ſtranger to its future deſignation, and to the element, for which its oily feathers, and web-like feet, are formed. Inſtincts analogous to theſe, operate, with equal energy, on the vegetable tribe. A ſeed contains a *germ*, or plant in miniature, and a *radicle*, or little root, intended by nature to ſupply it with nouriſhment. If the ſeed be ſown in an inverted

poſition,

poſition, ſtill each part purſues its proper direction. The *plumula* riſes upwards, and the *radicle* ſtrikes downward, into the ground. A hop-plant, turning round a pole, follows the courſe of the ſun, from ſouth to weſt, and ſoon dies, when forced into an oppoſite line of motion: But remove the obſtacle, and the plant will quickly return to its ordinary poſition. The branches of a honey-ſuckle ſhoot out longitudinally, till they become unable to bear their own weight; and then ſtrengthen themſelves, by changing their form into a ſpiral: When they meet with other living branches, of the ſame kind, they coaleſce, for mutual ſupport, and one ſpiral turns to the right, and the other to the left; thus ſeeking, by an inſtinctive impulſe, ſome body on which to climb, and increaſing the probability of finding one, by the diverſity of their courſe: For if the auxiliary branch be dead, the other uniformly winds itſelf round, from the right to the left *(c)*.

These examples, of the inſtinctive œconomy of vegetables, have been purpoſely taken from ſubjects familiar to our daily obſervation. But the plants of warmer climates, were we ſufficiently acquainted with them, would probably furniſh better illuſtrations of this acknowledged power of animality: And I ſhall briefly recite

(c) Lord Kaims's Gentleman Farmer.

the

the hiſtory of a very curious exotic, which has been delivered to us from good authority; and confirmed by the obſervations of ſeveral European botaniſts.

THE *Dionæa Muſcipula* is a native of North Carolina. Its leaves are numerous, inclining to bend downwards, and placed in a circular order: They are jointed, and ſucculent: The upper joint conſiſts of two lobes, each of which is ſemi-oval in its form, with a margin furniſhed with ſtiff hairs, which embrace each other, when they cloſe from any irritation. The ſurfaces of theſe lobes are covered with ſmall red glands, which probably ſecrete ſome ſweet liquor, tempting to the taſte, but fatal to the lives of inſects: For, the moment the poor animal alights upon theſe parts, the two lobes riſe up, graſp it forcibly, lock the rows of ſpines together, and ſqueeze it to death: And, leſt the ſtruggles for life ſhould diſengage the inſect, thus entangled, three ſmall ſpines are fixed amongſt the glands, near the middle of each lobe, which effectually put an end to all its efforts: Nor do the lobes open again, while the dead animal continues there. The diſſolution of its ſubſtance, therefore, is ſuppoſed by naturaliſts, to conſtitute part of the nouriſhment of the plant. But as the diſcriminative power of inſtinct is always limited, and proceeds with a blind

blind uniformity when put into exertion, the plant closes its leaves as forcibly, if stimulated by a straw or pin, as by the body of an insect; nor does it expand them again, till the extraneous substance is withdrawn *(d)*.

III. If the facts and observations, which have been adduced, furnish any presumptive proof of the instinctive power of vegetables, it will necessarily follow, that they must be endued with some degree of SPONTANEITY. For the impulse to discriminate and to prefer, is an actual exertion of that principle, however obscure the consciousness or the feeling may be, with which it is accompanied: And such volition presupposes an innate perception, both of what is consonant, and of what is injurious to the constitution of the individual, or species directed by it. But it is the design of this little Essay, rather to investigate nature, than to appeal to metaphysical considerations: I shall proceed, therefore, to point out a few of those phænomena, in the vegetable kingdom, which indicate spontaneity.

Several years ago, whilst engaged in a course of experiments to ascertain the influence of fixed air on vegetation, the following fact repeatedly occurred to me. A sprig of mint, suspended by the root, with the head downwards, in the middle

(d) See the Annual Register for 1775, p. 93.

middle glaſs veſſel of the machine for preparing mephitic water, continued to thrive vigorouſly, without any other *pabulum*, than what was ſupplied by the ſtream of *gas*, to which it was expoſed. In twenty four hours, the ſtem formed into a curve, the head became erect, and gradually aſcended towards the mouth of the veſſel; thus producing, by ſucceſſive efforts, a new and unuſual configuration of its parts. Such exertions in the ſprig of mint, to rectify its inverted poſition, and to remove from a foreign, to its natural element, ſeem to evince volition to avoid what was evil, and to recover what had been experienced to be good. If a plant, in a garden-pot, be placed in a room, which has no light, except from a hole in the wall, it will ſhoot towards the hole, paſs through it into the open air, and then vegetate upwards, in its proper direction. Lord Kaims relates, that, "amongſt the ruins of New Abbey, formerly a "monaſtery in Galloway, there grows on the "top of a wall, a plane tree, twenty feet high. "Straitened for nouriſhment, in that barren "ſituation, it ſeveral years ago directed roots "down the ſide of the wall, till they reached "the ground, ten feet below: And now, the "nouriſhment it afforded to theſe roots, during "the time of deſcending, is amply repaid; "having every year, ſince that time, made "vigorous

"vigorous ſhoots. From the top of the wall, to "the ſurface of the earth, theſe roots have not "thrown out a ſingle fibre, but are now united "into a pretty thick hard root(e)."

THE regular movement, by which the ſun-flower preſents its ſplendid diſk to the ſun, has been known to naturaliſts, and celebrated by poets, both of ancient and modern times. Ovid founds upon it a beautiful ſtory; and Thomſon deſcribes it, as an attachment of love to the celeſtial luminary.

"But one, the lofty follower of the ſun,
"Sad when he ſets, ſhuts up her yellow leaves,
"Drooping all night; and when he warm returns,
"Points her enamour'd boſom to his ray."

Summer, line 216.

IV. NATURE has wiſely proportioned the POWERS of MOTION, to the diverſified neceſſities of the beings endued with them. Corallines and Seapens are fixed to a ſpot, becauſe all their wants may be there ſupplied. The Oyſter, during the afflux of the tide, opens to admit the water, lying with the hollow ſhell downwards: But when the ebb commences, it turns on the other ſide; thus providing, by an inconſiderable movement, for the reception of its proper nutriment; and, afterwards, diſcharging what is ſuper-

(e) Gentleman Farmer.

ſluous.

fluous *(f)*. Mr. Miller, in his late account of the iſland of Sumatra, mentions a ſpecies of coral, which the inhabitants have miſtaken for a plant, and have denominated the Lalan-lout, or ſea-graſs. It is found in ſhallow bays, where it appears like a ſtraight ſtick, but when touched, withdraws itſelf into the ſand *(g)*. Now, if ſelf-moving faculties, like theſe, indicate animality, can ſuch a diſtinction be denied to vegetables, poſſeſſed of them in an equal, or ſuperior degree? The water-lily, be the pond deep or ſhallow in which it grows, puſhes up its flower-ſtems, till they reach the open air, that the *farina fecundans* may perform, without injury, its proper office. About ſeven in the morning, the ſtalk erects itſelf, and the flowers riſe above the ſurface of the water: In this ſtate they continue till four in the afternoon, when the ſtalk becomes relaxed, and the flowers ſink and cloſe. The motions of the ſenſitive plant have been long noticed with admiration, as exhibiting the moſt obvious ſigns of perceptivity. And, if we admit ſuch motions, as *criteria* of a like power, in other beings, to attribute them, in this inſtance, to mere mechaniſm, actuated ſolely by external impulſe, is to deviate from the ſoundeſt rule

(f) Sprat's Hiſtory of the Royal Society.

(g) Philoſoph. Tranſact. vol. LXVIII. p. 178.

of philoſophizing, which directs us not to multiply cauſes, when the effects appear to be the ſame. Neither will the laws of electricity better ſolve the phænomena of this animated vegetable: For its leaves are equally affected by the contact of electric, and non-electric bodies; ſhew no change in their ſenſibility, whether the atmoſphere be dry or moiſt; and inſtantly cloſe when the vapour of volatile alkali, or the fumes of burning ſulphur are applied to them. The powers of chemical *ſtimuli*, to produce contractions in the fibres of this plant, may perhaps lead ſome philoſophers, to refer them to the *vis inſita*, or irritability, which they aſſign to certain parts of organized matter, totally diſtinct from, and independent of, any ſentient energy. But the hypotheſis is evidently a ſoleciſm, and refutes itſelf. For the preſence of irritability can only be proved by the experience of irritations, and the idea of irritation involves in it that of feeling.

But there is a ſpecies of the order of *Decandria*, which conſtantly and uniformly exerts a ſelf-moving power, uninfluenced either by chemical *ſtimuli*, or by any external impulſe whatſoever. This curious ſhrub, which was unknown to Linnæus, is a native of the Eaſt Indies, but has been cultivated in ſeveral botanical gardens here. I had an opportunity of examining it, in in the collection of the late Dr. Brown. It is trifolious, grows to the height of four feet, and produces, in autumn, yellow flowers. The lateral leaves are smaller than those at the extremity of the stalk; and, all day long, they are continually moving either upwards, downwards, or horizontally in the segment of a circle. The last motion is performed by the twisting of the foot stalks: Whilst one leaf is rising, its associate is generally descending; but the motion downwards is quicker and more irregular, than the motion upwards, which is steady and uniform. These movements are observable, during the space of twenty-four hours, in the leaves of a branch lopped off from the shrub, and kept in water. If, from any obstacle, the motion be retarded, upon the removal of that obstacle, it is resumed with a greater degree of velocity *(b)*. I cannot better comment on this wonderful degree of vegetable animation, than in the words of Cicero. *Inanimum est omne quod pulsu agitatur externo; quod autem est animal, id motu cietur interiore et suo.*

I HAVE thus attempted, with the brevity prescribed by the laws of this Society, to extend our views of animated nature; to gratify the mind with the contemplation of multiplied ac-

(b) See Encyclopædia Britannica, Art. HEDYSARUM.

ceſſions to the general aggregate of felicity; and to exalt our conceptions of the wiſdom, power, and beneficence of God. In an undertaking, never yet accompliſhed, diſappointment can be no diſgrace: In one, directed to ſuch noble objects, the motives are a juſtification, independently of ſucceſs. Truth, indeed, obliges me to acknowledge, that I review my ſpeculations with much diffidence; and that, I dare not preſume to expect they will produce any permanent conviction in others, becauſe I experience an inſtability of opinion in myſelf. For again to uſe the language of Tully, *Neſcio quomodo, dum lego, aſſentior; cùm poſui librum, aſſenſio omnis illa elabitur.*—But this ſcepticiſm is perhaps to be aſcribed to the influence of habitual preconceptions, rather than to a deficiency of reaſonable proof. For beſides the various arguments which have been advanced, in favour of vegetable perceptivity, it may be further urged, that the hypotheſis recommends itſelf, by its conſonance to thoſe higher analogies of nature, which lead us to conclude, that the greateſt poſſible ſum of happineſs exiſts in the univerſe. The bottom of the ocean is overſpread with plants, of the moſt luxuriant magnitude. Immenſe regions of the earth are covered with perennial foreſts. Nor are the Alps, or the Andes, deſtitute of herbage, though buried in depths of ſnow. And can it it be imagined, that ſuch profuſion of life ſubſiſts without the leaſt ſenſation or enjoyment? Let us rather, with humble reverence, ſuppoſe, that vegetables participate, in ſome low degree, of the common allotment of vitality: And that our great Creator hath apportioned good, to all living things, "in number, weight, and meaſure *(i)*."

Supplement *to the foregoing* Paper; *containing further Obſervations on the* Sensitive Plant.

In the ſpeculations, concerning the perceptive power of vegetables, which were read before this

(i) It has been eſtimated, that our globe contains 20,000 ſpecies of vegetables; 3000 of worms; 12,000 of inſects; 200 of amphibious animals; 2,600 of fiſhes; 550 of birds; and 200 of quadrupeds. (Vid. Linn. Amœnit. Academ. and Stillingfleet's Miſcellaneous Tracts, p. 125). A calculation like this, it is evident, muſt be very defective; becauſe founded on paſt diſcoveries in a ſcience, which is now in a ſtate of rapid progreſſion.—"The great, the pious Mr. Ray," ſays Mr. Pennant, in a late work, (Index to Buffon's Ornithologie) "could not pronounce, that there were more than five hundred known ſpecies of birds; *M. Briſſon* has enlarged the liſt to above fourteen hundred; but our *Engliſh* ornithologiſt (Mr. *Latham)* deſcribes, with exactneſs, near two thouſand five hundred; which, with the varieties included in the *Synopſis*, and in the *Supplement*, may probably exceed 3,000."—Future acceſſions, both of plants and animals, with reſpect to number, may produce no material changes in their relative proportions.

 Society

Society laſt ſpring, I obſerved, that the motions of the ſenſitive plant are not to be explained by the laws of electricity. For its leaves are alike affected by the contact of electric and non-electric bodies; ſhew the ſame ſenſibility whether the atmoſphere be dry or moiſt; and inſtantly cloſe when certain chemical *ſtimuli*, ſuch as the vapour of vol. alkali, or the fumes of burning ſulphur, are applied to them. Theſe concluſions were founded on the recollection of experiments which I made more than twenty years ago. But the Abbé Bertholon de St. Lazane, in a late treatiſe on the electricity of vegetables, has adopted an oppoſite hypotheſis, and adduced the following trials in ſupport of it. When the ſenſitive plant, ſays he, is touched with a piece of poliſhed metal, terminated at each end by a round knob, its leaves ſhrink back and ſhut. When it is touched with a piece of glaſs, of the ſame form, it remains inſenſible. But if this piece of glaſs be electrified, and the plant be touched with it in this ſtate, the leaves inſtantly cloſe themſelves. Hence he infers, that the plants called *Mimoſæ* are endued with a much greater portion of electrical fluid than others; that this fluid eſcapes when touched by a foreign body, capable of conveying it away; and that they ſhrink by being thus deprived

deprived of what is eſſential to their health and vigour *(k)*.

I HAVE lately procured a ſenſitive plant, with the deſign of repeating the Abbé's experiments. But at the preſent ſeaſon of the year, I find this vegetable in a very languid ſtate; ſo that my trials have not afforded me much ſatisfaction. I could not, however, perceive any difference, whether the leaves were touched with a piece of poliſhed iron, or a ſtick of ſealing wax. And the following well authenticated facts, ſeem to refute the Abbé's hypotheſis, concerning the electrical œconomy of this plant.

I. THE branches of the ſenſitive plant have two motions, the one natural, the other artificial. By the firſt, it progreſſively increaſes, in the morning, the angle which it forms with the ſtem, and retreats in the ſame gradual manner, in the afternoon. By the ſecond, it contracts its leaves, when forcibly touched or ſhaken.

II. THE ſenſibility of the plant ſeems, chiefly, to reſide in the articulation of the branches of the common foot ſtalk, or of the particular foot ſtalk of each wing.

III. No motion enſues from cautiouſly piercing the branch with a needle, or other ſharp inſtrument.

(k) SEE Abbé Bertholon de St. Lazane Sur l'Electricité des Végétaux: Alſo Appendix to Monthly Review, vol. XVII. p. 135.

IV. A STROKE, or an irritation, produces a more forcible effect than an incision, or even an entire section.

V. A SLIGHT irritation only acts upon the neighbouring parts, and extends its influence according to its force.

VI. PLUNGING the plant in water seems to have no other effect than that of diminishing its vigour.

VII. A PIECE of wax, strongly electrified, made the leaves of the sensitive plant close quickly, by attracting them to it with considerable force.

VIII. THE motions of the sensitive plant are owing to a strong contraction. Each foot stalk seems to be terminated with a kind of joint, on which the leaves turn, with surprizing facility *(l)*.

NOVEMBER 9, 1784.

(l) Consult Milnes's Botanical Dictionary; the Encyclopædia Britannica; and Whytt on Vital Motions.

ESSAY

ESSAY IV.

FACTS AND QUERIES

RELATIVE TO

ATTRACTION AND REPULSION.

To the LITERARY and PHILOSOPHICAL SOCIETY of MANCHESTER *(a)*.

I COMMUNICATED to you, a few weeks ago, ſome curious and valuable obſervations, on the phænomena which take place between oil and water, tranſmitted to me by my learned and very ingenious friend Dr. Wall, of Oxford. My engagements deprived me of the pleaſure and inſtruction of attending their diſcuſſion, in the ſociety: And, ſolicitous to recover what I have loſt, I truſt you will indulge me with permiſſion to recall your attention to the ſubject, by the recital of a few miſcellaneous facts and inquiries, which the peruſal of that paper ſuggeſted to my mind.

(a) INSERTED in the Memoirs of the Literary and Philoſophical Society of Mancheſter, vol. II. p. 429.

I. If a glaſs tumbler, containing equal parts of water and of oil, in ſuch quantity as to occupy two thirds of it, be ſuſpended by a cord, and ſwung backwards and forwards, the oil will remain perfectly ſmooth and undiſturbed, whilſt the water below is in violent commotion. But if the oil be poured out, and its place ſupplied with water, the fluid will remain perfectly tranquil, throughout the whole veſſel, although the ſame motion be given to it as before. I have frequently repeated this experiment, and have ſometimes varied it, by ſubſtituting rectified ſpirit of wine, in the place of water. The oil then, being the heavier fluid, becomes agitated, whilſt the ſpirit remains at reſt. Dr. Franklin, who firſt noticed this ſingular phænomenon, informs us, that he ſhewed it to a number of ingenious perſons. "Thoſe," ſays he, "who are but "ſlightly acquainted with the principles of "hydroſtatics, &c. are apt to fancy, immedi-"ately, that they underſtand it, and readily "attempt to explain it: But their explanations "have been different, and, to me, not very "intelligible. Others more deeply ſkilled in "thoſe principles, ſeem to wonder at it, and "promiſe to conſider it. And I think it is "worth conſidering. For a new appearance, if "it cannot be explained by our old principles, "may afford us new ones, of uſe perhaps in "explaining

"explaining ſome other obſcure parts of natural "knowledge *(b)*." It is with diffidence, I offer as a conjecture, that the fact in queſtion, may ariſe from a *repulſive power*, ſubſiſting between the particles of oil and water, and depending, poſſibly, on the vibrations of that ſubtle æther, which Sir Iſaac Newton ſuppoſes to pervade all bodies. For, when this æther is excited into motion, by percuſſion or agitation, its elaſtic force is augmented, becauſe it becomes denſer in the pulſes of its vibrations, than in a quieſcent ſtate *(c)*. But in propoſing this hypotheſis, I may perhaps be chargeable with the paradoxical opinion of a celebrated French philoſopher, M. Fontenelle, who aſſerts, that if there be more than one way of accounting for any appearances in nature, there is a general preſumption, that they proceed from cauſes, which are leaſt obvious and familiar. I ſhall not, therefore, at preſent, enlarge upon this point, as it would anticipate what may be better urged, in our ſubſequent converſation. But the facts, above recited, furniſh a preſumption, that the effect of oily ſubſtances, on the cryſtallization of ſalt, is, in part,

(b) DR. FRANKLIN's Letters and Papers on Philoſophical Subjects, p. 438.

(c) ON the properties of this Æther, conſult Dr. Bryan Robinſon's Works, *paſſim*.

owing

owing to a mechanical cauſe. At Droitwich, it is the practice, as appears by Dr. Wall's quotation from the Hiſtory of Worceſterſhire, to throw, into the brine pan, a piece of reſin, about the ſize of a pea, to produce a finer granulation. The more reſin they uſe, the ſmaller will be the grain of the ſalt; and if a lump, of the ſize of two walnuts, were put into the pan, the particles of ſalt would be ſo minute as not to be capable of ſubſiding. Reſin, butter, or tallow, when liquefied by the heat of the boiling brine, float upon its ſurface, and will remain perfectly ſmooth and undiſturbed, whilſt the water, beneath, may be put into ſtrong agitation, by the action of the fire. Such agitation muſt break down the cryſtals of ſalt, as they ſhoot; and conſequently, only ſmall granules will be produced.

II. Every one has experienced the ſuffocating effects of air, loaded with the *effluvia* of burnt greaſe, or the ſnuff of a lamp. When ſuch fumes are inſpired, there is the ſenſation of a conflict in the lungs, which eſſentially differs from what is felt, on breathing either fixed or inflammable air. And is not the moſt eaſy ſolution of it, to ſuppoſe, that the air quits the oily, to unite with the watery vapours, which are brought into contiguity, by this action of the animal œconomy; and that a ſtrong repulſion ſucceeds? "For, as in algebra, where "affirmative

"affirmative quantities vaniſh and ceaſe, there "negative ones begin, ſo, in mechanics, where "attraction ceaſes, there a repulſive power ought "to ſucceed," according to the doctrine of Sir Iſaac Newton. It is, alſo, an axiom, laid down by this great philoſopher, that "to the ſame "natural effects, we muſt always aſſign, as "far as poſſible, the ſame cauſes." I ſhall therefore proceed to illuſtrate this ſubject, by other more deciſive examples of *repulſion*; after premiſing a few obſervations on that ſpecies of *attraction*, which appears to be the cônverſe of it.

III. THAT the particles of homogeneous bodies have an affinity to, and conſequently attract each other, is conſonant both to analogy and obſervation. Fluids manifeſt this property, by their diſpoſition to aſſume a globular figure, and by the ruſhing together of theſe globules, when brought within their reciprocal ſphere of activity. A ſimilar attraction ſubſiſts between heterogeneous ſubſtances, which is diſtinct from that of *coheſion*, as it partakes of an *elective* nature, and yet cannot be deemed *chemical*, becauſe no combination is produced by it, ſo intimate, as to manifeſt any change of properties. This may be illuſtrated by the increaſe of power, in the ſuſpenſion of weights, which a hair acquires, by being moiſtened with different liquids. For ſuch additional ſtrength is not proportioned, preciſely, precifely, to the tenacity of the liquid employed; and probably fubfifts in a duplicate ratio, compounded of the affinity which the parts of the liquid bear to each other, and to the minuteft fibres of the hair. The particles of water attract one another more ftrongly, than they attract polifhed wood or ftone; whilft, on the contrary, they are lefs forcibly attracted by each other than by glafs. This is evinced by the common experiment with capillary tubes. For the water, which afcends, muft have quitted the contact of the water left behind, contrary to their mutual affinity, as well as to the law of gravitation. The particles of quickfilver, like water, are attracted by glafs. For if a fmall globule of this metal be laid upon unfullied paper, and touched with a piece of clean polifhed glafs, the quickfilver will adhere to the latter, in preference to the former, and may be drawn away with it. But the relation of mercury to glafs is of inferior force, to that which fubfifts between its own particles. This will appear by dipping a bent tube, open at both ends, into a veffel, filled with quickfilver, which will enter into the tube, but ftand within it, below the furface of the mercury, at a depth, proportionate to the diameter of the tube *(d)*. It is unneceffary to

(d) Confult Dr. Jurin's Experiments, Philofophical Tranfactions, No. 363; alfo Cotes's Hydroftatical Lectures p. 231.

adduce further inſtances of this attraction; and I ſhall endeavour to ſhew, that where it does not ſubſiſt, a repulſive power apparently takes place. This, according to the laws of optics, has been deduced from the globules of rain, which lie on the leaves of colewort, whoſe luſtre and mobility are ſo ſtriking to the eye. For, on a cloſe inſpection of them, it is found, that the luſtre is produced by a copious reflection of light, from their flattened inferior parts. It has alſo been further obſerved, that when a drop rolls along a leaf, which has been wetted, its brightneſs diſappears, and the green leaf, before hardly diſcernible, is now ſeen clearly through it. From theſe facts it is inferred, that the globule does not touch the plant; but that it is ſuſpended at ſome diſtance, in the air, by the force of a repulſive power; becauſe there could not be any copious reflection of white light, from its under ſurface, unleſs a real interval ſubſiſted between that ſurface and the plant *(e)*. This hypotheſis accounts for the volubility of the drop, and for its leaving no trace of moiſture, where it rolls. From the like reaſoning it hath been concluded, that when a poliſhed needle is made to lie on water, it is not in contact with

(e) See Newton's Optics, Query 29. Alſo the Edinburgh Phyſical and Literary Eſſays, vol. II. p. 25.

that

that fluid, but forms, by repulſion, a bed, whoſe concavity is much larger than its own bulk. Hence it is readily conceived, how the needle ſwims upon a liquid, lighter than itſelf; ſince the quantity of water, diſplaced by it, may be equal to its weight. Can it be philoſophical, to attribute ſuch a phænomenon to the tenacity of water, or to the attraction ſubſiſting between its particles?

IV. The attractions and repulſions between thoſe exhalations that are termed DEW, and certain ſubſtances expoſed to them, are ſtill more remarkable, than the facts which have been already recited. M. Muſſchenbroek placed different bodies, for the reception of theſe vapours, on the terrace of the obſervatory at Utrecht, and found that ſome caught them abundantly, others only in a ſmall quantity, but that a third ſort repelled them altogether *(f)*. M. du Fay, of the French Academy, repeated theſe experiments, and fully proved that, whilſt the dew fell copiouſly into veſſels of glaſs, not the leaſt moiſture was apparent in veſſels of poliſhed metal, contiguous to them. To be aſſured whether the difference was always the ſame, in all circumſtances, between vitrified ſubſtances and metals, he ſet a China ſaucer in the middle of a ſilver

(f) Introd. ad Philoſ. Nat. vol. II. p. 990.

plate,

plate, and, on one ſide, adjoining to it, put a ſilver veſſel, very like the ſaucer, upon a China plate. The former, viz. the China ſaucer, was covered with dew, although the plate, which ſpread four inches around it, had not a ſingle drop. The China plate, alſo, received the dew, whilſt the ſilver veſſel, that was in the middle, remained as dry, as when it was firſt expoſed.

THE ſame ingenious philoſopher endeavoured to aſcertain, whether a China ſaucer, ſet upon a plate of metal, in the manner above deſcribed, did not receive more dew, than it would have done, if expoſed quite alone. To accompliſh this deſign, he took two watch cryſtals, of equal dimenſions, and placed the one upon a plate of ſilver, the other upon a plate of China, each with its concavity uppermoſt. That which was upon the ſilver plate, he ſurrounded with a ferrel, of the ſame metal, well poliſhed, that no watery particles might attach themſelves to the convex ſurface of the glaſs. Thus circumſtanced, he expoſed the cryſtals, ſeveral days ſucceſſively, in a proper ſituation, and always found five or ſix times more dew in that, which was on the China plate, than in the other placed on ſilver: And this may be regarded as a preſumptive proof, that the moiſture repelled from the metal, was attracted by the China. That there ſubſiſted ſuch a repulſion, is confirmed by the following obſervation of M. du Fay, with regard to the

 cryſtal

cryſtal on the ſilver plate. He informs us, that the ſmall quantity of dew on the inſide, was only near the centre, in minute drops; and that, round the border, there was a ſpace of five or ſix lines, perfectly dry, towards which the drops regularly decreaſed, in magnitude; as if the ſilver ferrel had *driven away* the dew from that part of the glaſs, which was contiguous to it. Theſe experiments were repeated thirty times, with invariable ſucceſs *(g)*. And Dr. Watſon, now Biſhop of Landaff, has lately confirmed them, by ſome very curious trials, of a ſimilar kind, made to determine the quantity of vapours which aſcend, in a given ſpace, from the ſurface of the earth. " By means of a little bees wax," ſays he, " I faſtened a half crown very near, but " not quite contiguous to the ſide of the glaſs; " and ſetting the glaſs, with its mouth down- " wards, on the graſs, it preſently became " covered with vapour, except that part of it, " which was near to the half crown. Not only " the half crown itſelf, was free from vapour, " but it had hindered any from ſettling on the " glaſs, which was near it, for there was a little " ring of glaſs ſurrounding the half crown, to " the diſtance of a quarter of an inch, which " was quite dry, as well as that part of the glaſs, " which was immediately under the half crown; " it ſeemed as if the ſilver had repelled the water

(g) Vid. Hiſt. de l'Acad. des Scienc. 1749.

" to

"to that diſtance. A large red wafer had the "ſame effect as the half crown; it was neither "wetted itſelf, nor was the ring of glaſs, con- "tiguous to it, wetted. A circle of white paper "produced the ſame effect, ſo did ſeveral other "ſubſtances, which it would be tedious to "enumerate (*h*)."

Do not the inſtances of repulſion, here adduced, with various others, which may perhaps be recollected and noticed by the Gentlemen preſent, warrant us to conclude, that this principle is a powerful agent, in the operations of nature? To this cauſe, the air we breathe owes, probably, its exiſtence and elaſticity; the light, which illuminates our globe, its rapid motions and diverſified inflections; and fire, its genial, expanſile, and animating energy. Is it, therefore, conſiſtent with analogy, to exclude repulſion from that branch of phyſics, which chemiſtry comprehends? The ſubject certainly merits further inveſtigation: And I ſhall ſtate, to my friend Dr. Wall, the facts and queries, which I have now laid before this Society; that he may communicate to us ſuch limitations or confirmations of his doctrine, as an attentive review of it may ſuggeſt, to his ingenuous and philoſophic mind.

(*h*) Watſon's Chemical Eſſays, vol. III. p. 64.

ESSAY V.

A NARRATIVE OF THE

SUFFERINGS OF A COLLIER,

Who was confined more than ſeven Days, without SUSTENANCE, and expoſed to the CHOKE-DAMP, in a COAL PIT not far from MANCHESTER;

WITH OBSERVATIONS ON THE

EFFECTS OF FAMINE;

On the MEANS *of* ALLEVIATING *them*; *and on the* ACTION *of* FOUL AIR *on the* HUMAN BODY *(a)*.

IN compliance with the requeſt of this Society, I have obtained an authentic account of the caſe of the unfortunate man, who was ſo long confined in a coal pit at Hurſt, near Aſhton-under-line. My information, concerning him, has been communicated by Mr. John Lees, of Clarksfield, in that neighbourhood, a Gentleman of probity and good ſenſe, who him-

(a) INSERTED in the Memoirs of the Mancheſter Society, vol. II. p. 467.

ſelf

ſelf very humanely aſſiſted the poor ſufferer, and collected in perſon, or received from thoſe who attended him till his death, the intelligence with which he has favoured me.

On Saturday the fourth of December, 1784, about eight o'clock in the morning, Thomas Travis, a collier, aged twenty-ſeven, deſcended into the pit at Hurſt, which is ninety yards in depth; and ſeveral other workmen were in readineſs to follow him. But ſoon after he had reached the bottom, the ſides of the pit fell in, and he was cut off from all ſupplies of the external air. The quantity of earth was ſo large, that it required ſix days to remove it: And on Thurſday, when the paſſage was completed, the foulneſs of the vapours prevented any one, for ſome time, from venturing into the works. On Friday, ſeveral men entered the coal-mine; but not finding Travis, they conjectured that he had attempted to dig his way into another pit, at no great diſtance. They followed him by the traces of his working; and on Saturday afternoon, about four o'clock, he heard them, and implored their ſpeedy aſſiſtance. When they reached him, he was laid upon his belly, and raiſing his head, he looked at the men, and addreſſed one of them by his name. But his eyes were ſo ſwoln and protruded, that they were ſhocked with the appearance of them; and they prevailed upon him to ſuffer a handkerchief to be tied round his head, aſſigning, as a reaſon, that the light might prove dangerous and offenſive to him. *Sal volatile* was then held to his noſtrils, and ſoon afterwards he complained of the handkerchief, and deſired them to remove it. They complied with his requeſt; but his eyes were then ſunk in their ſockets, and he was unable to diſtinguiſh the candle, though held directly before him. Nor did he ever afterwards perceive the leaſt glimmering of light. He aſked for ſomething to drink; and was ſupplied with water gruel, that had been previouſly provided, of which he took a table ſpoonful, every ten or fifteen minutes. When the men firſt diſcovered him, his hands and feet were extremely cold, and no pulſe could be felt at the wriſt. But after he had taſted the gruel, and ſmelled at the *ſal volatile*, the pulſation of the artery became ſenſible, and grew ſtronger when they had rubbed him, and covered him with blankets. He now complained of pain in his head and limbs, and ſaid, his back felt as if it had been broken. Two men lay by his ſides, to communicate warmth to him, he put his hands into their boſoms; expreſſed his ſenſe of its being comfortable; and ſlept, when he was not rouſed to take nouriſhment. In this ſituation he he remained ſeveral hours, till they had completed a road for his conveyance out of the pit. Whilſt they were carrying him, he had a motion to make water and to go to ſtool, but had not ſufficient power to accompliſh either. At one o'clock on Sunday morning, he was brought to his own houſe; put into bed, well covered, and fed with chicken broth. But his weakneſs rendered him indifferent to nouriſhment. He continued to doze and ſleep; and notwithſtanding his pulſe ſeemed at firſt to increaſe in vigour, it became quick about five o'clock, when he warned them of his approaching end, and expired, without a ſtruggle, in a few minutes. Though Travis had been aſthmatic for many years, his reſpiration was remarked to be clear and eaſy, under the circumſtances above deſcribed. He remained perfectly ſenſible till his death; but had no accurate idea of the duration of his confinement in the pit: For on being interrogated concerning this point, he eſtimated the time to have been only two days, yet added, that he thought thoſe days were very long.

As the foregoing account is defective in ſome intereſting particulars, I have applied to Mr. Lees for further information; and ſhall lay before the Society the ſubſtance of the anſwers, which he has returned to my ſeveral queries.

1. I INQUIRED, what food Travis had taken, during the ſpace of twenty-four hours, before he went into the coal pit; and have been informed, that, on Friday morning, he eat a meſs of water pottage and milk, to his breakfaſt; had roaſted beef and potatoes to his dinner; broth and pudding to his ſupper; and on the Saturday morning, juſt before his deſcent into the coal mine, a cup of broth and a piece of bread and cheeſe.

2. IT is not known whether he had any evacuations in the coal pit, no marks of them having been diſcovered.

3. THERE is no doubt that he could ſee, at the time when he was found, as he gave aſſurances of it to the men, notwithſtanding the tumefaction and protruſion of his eyes.

4. THE compaſs of the cavity which he had dug, and where he was laid upon his belly, at the time when the men reached him, was three yards in length, and two in width. The ſtratum of coal is about two feet thick. There was a communication between the place where he was confined, and another pit. But as the paſſage was eight yards long, and in no part more than eight or ten inches wide, the mouth of the pit alſo, into which he had deſcended, being ſtopt, and the body of earth, through which he had dug, thrown behind him, no circulation of

of air could poſſibly take place. And the truth of this concluſion is evinced by the ſtate of the air, in the other pit, to which this paſſage led. For it was there ſo foul as to extinguiſh the candles, which the workmen carried down, in order to come at Travis by the way, which they denominate, the *air-gate(b).*

5. THE temperature of the air varies much in coal pits, even of the ſame depth. No thermometrical obſervations were made on the preſent occaſion; but the ſenſations of Travis ſeem to have indicated coldneſs; and his extremities never recovered their natural warmth. Moiſture always abounds in theſe mines.

6. THE weakneſs of Travis prevented him from giving any account of his ſufferings, either from hunger or thirſt. But it was obſerved that he was eager to drink, at the time when he was found.

(b) THE ventilation of this ſubterranean paſſage might, perhaps, have been expedited, and the *mephitis* almoſt inſtantly corrected, by carrying down into it buckets of water, and ſlaking in them a ſufficient quantity of freſh burnt quicklime. The hot ſteam, generated by this operation, it may be preſumed, would have diffuſed itſelf quickly through the whole cavity; the gas would have united with the aqueous vapour; been precipitated with it; and a current of atmoſpheric air would have ruſhed in to ſupply its place.

7. IT

7. It is certain that Travis had no provisions with him, in the coal mine; and that there was not any supply of water, except near the mouth of the pit; a place he must immediately have quitted, and to which he deprived himself of the power of returning, by throwing the earth behind him, in his progress. We may therefore presume, that he passed the whole seven days of his confinement, without either meat or drink.

This affecting catastrophe coincides, in a striking manner, with an observation of Hippocrates, *That most of those, who neither eat nor drink for seven days, die within that period. And that though they survive, so as afterwards to take nourishment, their former fasting will prove fatal to them (c).* Yet it is evident, that the remark of this faithful recorder of facts, was founded on experience too limited, to give it validity. For we have many well attested accounts of longer continued abstinence, without destruction to life. Sir William Hamilton, in his narrative of the earthquakes in Italy, A. D. 1783, mentions a girl, of sixteen years of age, who remained eleven days without food, under the ruins of a house at Oppido. She had a child in her arms, five or six months old, who

(c) Hippocrat. de Carnibus. sect. III.

died

died the fourth day. A light, through a ſmall chaſm, enabled her to aſcertain the time of her confinement, and ſhe gave a very clear relation of her ſufferings. When Sir William Hamilton ſaw her, ſhe did not appear to be in bad health, drank eaſily, but with difficulty ſwallowed any thing ſolid *(d)*. In caſes of this kind, is it not probable that the body may be ſupplied with fluids from the external air, by the exertion of ſome extraordinary powers in the lymphatic ſyſtem? Thus the negro, mentioned by Dr. Chalmers, who was gibbeted at Charleſtown, in March 1779, and had nothing given him afterwards, regularly voided every morning, till he died, a large quantity of urine *(e)*. The ſpring ſeaſon, in South Carolina, is attended with great nocturnal dews, which being imbibed by the pores of the ſkin, furniſhed the poor negro with a ſuperabundance of fluids in the night, and a ſufficiency to ſupport perſpiration in the day. I viſited, not long ſince, in conſultation with her kinſman Dr. Eaſon, an elderly lady, who laboured under a very ſevere lientery. Her evacuations, as often happens both in this diſeaſe and in the diabetes, far exceeded in quantity, the liquids which ſhe ſwallowed, or what could be aſcribed to the diſſolution of her ſolids.

(d) Phil. Tranſ. vol. LXXIII. p. 169.

(e) Chalmers on Fevers, p. 2.

During

During five or ſix days before her death, ſhe took no aliment whatever, and only occaſionally moiſtened her mouth, by putting her fingers into it, after they had been dipped in water. Yet ſhe diſcharged a pint of urine once in twenty-four hours. I am inclined to conjecture, that the moiſture of the coal pit was favourable to Travis; but how long he might have ſubſiſted under ſuch circumſtances, it is not poſſible to determine. It may however be preſumed, that his death was rather accelerated than retarded, by the changes and the hurry which he underwent.

In famine, life may be protracted with leſs pain and miſery, by a moderate allowance of water. For the acrimony and putrefaction of the humours are obviated by ſuch dilution, the ſmall veſſels are kept permeable, and the lungs are furniſhed with that moiſture, which is eſſential to the performance of their functions. Fantonus, a writer of reſpectable authority in the eſtimation of Morgagni, relates the hiſtory of a woman, who obſtinately refuſed to take any ſuſtenance, except twice, during the ſpace of fifty days, at the end of which period ſhe died *(f)*. But

(f) Morgagni de Sedibus et Cauſis Morborum. Epiſt. XXVII.

Sir William Blackstone (book IV. ch. 25.) ſpeaking of the Engliſh judgment of Penance, ſays, " that the " priſoner

But he adds, that ſhe uſed water, by way of drink, though in ſmall quantity. Redi, who made many experiments, (cruel and unjuſtifiable in my opinion) to aſcertain the effects of faſting on fowls, obſerved, that none were able to ſupport life beyond the ninth day, to whom drink was denied; whereas one, indulged with water, lived more than twenty days.

HIPPOCRATES has obſerved, that children are more affected by abſtinence than young perſons; theſe, more than the middle aged; and the middle aged, more than old men. Agreeably to this aphoriſm, Dante is ſaid, by his countryman Morgagni, to have framed the incidents in the affecting ſtory of Count Ugolino, a nobleman of Piſa, who was confined, with his four ſons, in the dungeon of a tower; the key of which being caſt into the river Arno, they were, in this horrible ſituation, ſtarved to death. And they are repreſented by the poet, as dying at different periods, according to their reſpective

" priſoner ſhall have no ſuſtenance, ſave only on the firſt day " three morſels of the worſt bread, and on the ſecond day " three draughts of ſtanding water; and, in this ſituation, " this ſhall be alternately his daily diet, till he dies." By a record of 35 Edward I. it is clearly proved, that the priſoner might then poſſibly ſubſiſt *forty days*, under this lingering puniſhment.

ages

ages *(g)*. Travis, being in the prime of life, was fitted to bear the extremities of want, better than he could have done in the ftate of adolefcence, when the body calls for conftant nutriment, to fupport its growth. But of what he felt we are left in uncertainty, as he declined, through weaknefs, to give any relation of it. There are conftitutions, which do not fuffer much pain from the calls of hunger. I have been informed, by a young phyfician from Geneva, that, when he was a ftudent at Montpelier, he fafted three nights and four days, with no other refrefhment than a pint of water daily. His hunger was keen, but never painful, during the firft and fecond days of his abftinence; and the two

(g) On reviewing the ftory of Count Ugolino, as related by Dante, in his thirty-third Canto, I find that Morgagni is miftaken in fuppofing the incidents of it conformable to the obfervation of Hippocrates. Nor is the poet to be condemned, as deviating from truth or nature; becaufe the power to endure famine muft depend no lefs upon the ftate of health and ftrength, than on the age of the fufferer. The following lines are copied from the tranflation of this Poem, by the Earl of Carlifle.

Now the fourth morning rofe; my eldeft child
Fell at his father's feet, in accent wild,
Struggling with pain, with his laft fleeting breath,
"Help me, my fire," he cried, and funk in death.
I faw the others follow one by one,
Heard their laft fcream, and their expiring groan.

following

following days, he perceived only a faintneſs, when he attempted either bodily or mental exertion: A ſenſe of coldneſs was diffuſed over his whole frame, but more particularly affected the extremities. His mind was in a very unuſual ſtate of puſillanimity; and he experienced a great tendency to tears, whenever he recollected the circumſtance, which had been the occaſion of his faſting. During the whole period, the alvine excretions were ſuppreſſed, but not thoſe by the kidney: And at the cloſe of it, his ſkin became tinged with a ſhade of yellow. The firſt food he took was veal broth, which had ſomething of an intoxicating effect, producing a glow of warmth, and raiſing his ſpirits, ſo as to render him aſhamed of his deſpondency. Perhaps in the caſe of Sextius Baculus, as recorded in the Commentaries of Cæſar *(b)*, the extraordinary courage and proweſs which he ſuddenly exerted, might be aided by the exhilarating effect of ſuſtenance, which, under ſuch circumſtances, it is probable he would no longer decline. The fact however evinces, that neither his ſickneſs nor the ſenſations of hunger had been ſo violent, as much to impair his ſtrength of body or vigour of mind. Pomponius Atticus, the celebrated friend of Cicero, who put a voluntary end to his

(b) De Bello Gallico, lib. VI.

life in the ſeventy-ſeventh year of his age, by refuſing all food, appears to have experienced eaſe from his diſorder, rather than any acute ſufferings, by famine *(i)*. From the former circumſtance it has been conjectured, that he did not wholly deny himſelf the uſe of water, or of ſome other diluent. But though a few examples of this kind may be adduced, we have the evidence of numerous melancholy facts to ſhew, that the preſſure of want is agonizing to the human frame. " I have talked," ſays an ingenious writer, " with the captain of a ſhip, who " was one of ſix, that endured it in its extremity, " and who was the only perſon that had not loſt " his ſenſes, when they received accidental relief. " He aſſured me his pains, at firſt, were ſo great, " as to be often tempted to eat a part of one of " the men who died, and which the reſt of his " crew, actually for ſome time, lived upon: He " ſaid, that during the continuance of this " paroxyſm, he found his pains inſupportable, " and was deſirous, at one time, of anticipating " that death, which he thought inevitable: But " his pains, he ſaid, gradually decreaſed, after the " ſixth day, (for they had water in the ſhip, which

(i) Sic cum biduò cibo ſe abſtinuiſſet, ſubito febris deceſſit, leviorque, morbus eſſe cæpit: Tamen propoſitum nihilo ſecius peregit. Itaque die quinto, poſtquam id conſilium inierat, deceſſit. Corn. Nepos in Vit. Pomp. Attic.

" kept

"kept them alive ſo long,) and then he was in "a ſtate rather of languor, than deſire; nor did he "much wiſh for food, except when he ſaw others "eating; and that for a while revived his appe-"tite, though with diminiſhed importunity. The "latter part of the time, when his health was "almoſt deſtroyed, a thouſand ſtrange images "roſe upon, his mind; and every one of his "ſenſes began to bring him wrong information. "The moſt fragrant perfumes appeared to him "to have a fetid ſmell; and every thing he "looked at took a greeniſh hue, and ſometimes "a yellow. When he was preſented with food "by the ſhip's company, that took him and his "men up, four of whom died ſhortly after, he "could not help looking upon it with loathing "inſtead of deſire; and it was not, till after four "days, that his ſtomach was brought to its natu-"ral tone; when the violence of his appetite "returned, with a ſort of canine eagerneſs *(k)*."

To thoſe who, by their occupations, are expoſed to ſuch dreadful calamities, it is of ſerious importance to be inſtructed in the means of alleviating them. The American Indians are ſaid to uſe a compoſition of the juice of tobacco, and the ſhells of ſnails, cockles, and oyſters calcined, whenever they undertake a long journey, and

(k) See Goldſmith's Hiſtory of the Earth, vol. II. p. 126.

are likely to be deſtitute of proviſions. It is probable, the ſhells are not burnt into quicklime, but only ſo as to deſtroy their tenacity, and to render them fit for levigation. The maſs is dried, and formed into pills, of a proper ſize to be held between the gum and lip, which, being gradually diſſolved and ſwallowed, obtund the ſenſations both of hunger and of thirſt. Tobacco, by its narcotic quality, ſeems well adapted to counteract the uneaſy impreſſions, which the gaſtric juice makes on the nerves of the ſtomach, when it is empty: And the combination of teſtaceous powders with it may tend to correct the ſecretion that is ſuppoſed, by an eminent anatomiſt, to be the chief agent in digeſtion, and which, if not acid, is always united with acidity *(l)*. Certain at leaſt it is, that their operation is both grateful and ſalutary; for we find the luxurious inhabitants of the Eaſt Indies mix them with the betle nut, to the chewing of which they are univerſally and immoderately addicted. Perhaps ſuch abſorbents may be uſefully applied, both to divide the doſes, and to moderate the virulence of the tobacco. For, in the internal exhibition of this plant, much caution is required, as it produces ſickneſs, vertigo, cold clammy ſweats, and a train of other formidable ſymptoms, when taken in too

(l) See Mr. John Hunter's paper, on the digeſtion of the ſtomach after death. Philoſ. Tranſact. for 1772.

large

large a quantity. During the time of war, the impreſſed ſailors frequently bring on theſe maladies, that they may be admitted into the hoſpitals, and releaſed from ſervitude. It would be an eaſy and ſafe experiment to aſcertain the efficacy, and to adjuſt the ingredients of the Indian compoſition, which I have mentioned. And I am inclined to believe, that the trial would be, in ſome degree, ſucceſsful, becauſe I have repeatedly experienced, in the courſe of my profeſſional practice, that ſmoking tobacco gives relief, in thoſe habitual pains of the ſtomach, which appear to ariſe from the irritation of the gaſtric ſecretions. The like effect is ſometimes produced by increaſing the flow of ſaliva, and ſwallowing what is thus diſcharged *(m)*. And I have elſewhere related the caſe of a gentleman, who uſed to maſticate, many hours daily, a piece of lead, which, being neither hard, friable, nor offenſive to the palate, ſuited his purpoſe, as he thought, better than any other ſubſtance. He continued the cuſtom many years, deriving great eaſe from it, and ſuffering no ſenſible injury from the poiſonous quality of the metal. On

(m) A LADY, in this neighbourhood, was relieved of a chronic pain in the ſtomach, by chewing *amara dulcis*, after various other remedies had failed: And I have ſeen good effects from the *calamus aromaticus*, uſed in the ſame way.

 mentioning

mentioning this fact to a navy surgeon, he acquainted me, that the sailors, when in hot climates, are wont to mitigate thirst, by rolling a bullet in their mouths. A more innocent mean might be devised; but the efficacy of this evinces, that the salivary glands are, for a while, capable of furnishing a substitute for drink. When a scarcity of water occurs at sea, Dr. Franklin has advised, that the mariners should bathe themselves in tubs of salt-water: For, in pursuing the amusement of swimming, he observed that, however thirsty he was before immersion, he never continued so afterwards; and that, though he soaked himself several hours in the day, and several days successively, in salt-water, he perceived not, in consequence of it, the least taste of saltness in his mouth. He also further suggests, that the same good effect might perhaps be derived from dipping the sailor's apparel in the sea; and expresses a confidence, that no danger of catching cold would ensue.

To prevent the calamity of famine at sea, it has been proposed, that the powder of SALEP should constitute part of the provisions of every ship's company *(n)*. This powder, and portable soup, dissolved in boiling water, form a rich thick jelly; and an ounce of each of these articles fur-

(n) Lind on the Diseases of Hot Climates.

nishes one day's subsistence to a healthy, full grown man. Indeed, from the experiments which I have made on salep, I have reason to believe the supposition well founded, that it contains more nutritious matter, in proportion to its bulk, than any other vegetable production, now used as food (o). It has the property, also, of concealing the nauseous taste of salt-water; and consequently may be of great advantage at sea, when the stock of fresh water is so far consumed, that the mariners are put upon short allowance. By the same mucilaginous quality, it covers the offensiveness, and even, in some measure, corrects the acrimony, of salted and putrescent meats. But, as a preservative against hunger, salep would be most efficacious, combined with an equal weight of beef suet. By swallowing little balls of this lubricating compound, at proper intervals, the coats of the stomach would be defended from irritation: And as oils and mucilages are highly nutritive, of slow digestion, and indisposed to pass off by perspiration, they are peculiarly well adapted to support life, in small quantities. This composition is superior in simplicity, and perhaps equal in efficacy, to the following one, so much extolled by Avicenna, the celebrated Arabian physician; to whom we are indebted for the introduction of rhubarb, cassia, tamarinds, and

(o) See vol I. p. 288.

ſena, into the *Materia Medica.* "Take ſweet "almonds, and beef ſuet, of each one pound; of "the oil of violets two ounces; and of the roots "of marſh mallows one ounce: Bray theſe ingre- "dients together, in a mortar, and form the maſs "into boluſes, about the ſize of a common nut." Animal fat is ſingularly powerful in aſſuaging the moſt acute ſenſations of thirſt; as appears from the narrative of the ſufferings experienced by thoſe, who were confined in the black hole at Calcutta. A hundred and forty-ſix perſons, exhauſted by fatigue and military duty, were there thruſt together into a chamber of eighteen cubic feet, having only two windows, ſtrongly barred with iron, from which, in a cloſe ſultry night, and in ſuch a climate as that of Bengal, little or no circulation of freſh air could be enjoyed. In a few minutes, theſe unhappy wretches fell into ſo profuſe a perſpiration, that an idea can hardly be formed of it; and this was ſucceeded by a raging thirſt, which increaſed in proportion as the body was drained of its moiſture. Water! water! became the univerſal cry; and an old ſoldier on the outſide, through pity, furniſhed them with a few ſkinfulls of it. But theſe ſcanty ſupplies, like ſprinklings on the fire, ſerved only to feed and increaſe the flame. From this experience of its effects, Mr. Holwell,

Holwell, their chief, determined to drink no more; and kept his mouth moiſt, by ſucking the perſpiration out of his ſhirt ſleeves, and catching the drops as they fell from his head and face. You cannot imagine, ſays he, how unhappy I was, if any of them eſcaped me. He came into the priſon without his coat, the ſeaſon being too hot to bear it: and one of his miſerable companions, obſerving the expedient he had hit upon, of allaying his thirſt, robbed him, from time to time, of a conſiderable part of his ſtore. This plunderer, whom he found to be a young gentleman in the ſervice of the Eaſt India Company, afterwards acknowledged, that he owed his life to the many comfortable draughts, which he derived from him. Before Mr. Holwell adopted this mode of relief, he had attempted, in an ungovernable fit of thirſt, to drink his own urine: But it was ſo intenſely bitter, that a ſecond taſte could not be endured; whereas, he aſſures us, no Briſtol water could be more ſoft and pleaſant than his perſpiration *(p)*. And this, we may preſume, conſiſted chiefly of animal fat, melted by exceſſive heat, and exuding from the cellular membrane, through the pores of the ſkin.

Persons who have been accuſtomed to animal food, are ſoon reduced, when ſupplied only

(p) See Annual Regiſter for 1758, p. 278.

with the *farinacea*. Several years ago, to determine the comparative nutritive powers of different ſubſtances, an ingenious young phyſician, of my acquaintance, made a variety of experiments on himſelf, to which he unfortunately fell a ſacrifice. I have been informed, that he lived a month upon bread and water, and that, under this regimen of diet, he every day diminiſhed much in his weight. But laſt winter, a ſtudent of phyſic at Edinburgh, confined himſelf, for a longer ſpace of time, to a pint of milk, and half a pound of white bread daily: And he aſſures me, that he paſſed through the uſual labours of ſtudy and exerciſe, without feeling any decay of health or ſtrength, and without any ſenſible loſs of bulk *(q)*. The cutaneous, urinary, and alvine excretions were very ſcanty during the whole period; and the diſcharge of fæces occurred only once in a week. In this caſe, the oily and coagulable parts of the milk probably furniſhed a larger proportion of aliment, and at the ſame time contributed to check the waſte, by perſpiration and other diſcharges. For

(q) THE following fact, cited by Haller, ſhews the powers of milk, in ſmall quantities, to ſupport life; but does not aſcertain how far it ſupplies or obviates the waſte of the body. *Lactis in diem libra, tres feminæ, à nivis ruinâ obrutæ, per* 37 *dies vitam ſuſtentarunt.* HALLER. ELEMENT. PHYSIOLOG. vol. IV. p. 255.

oleaginous

oleaginous ſubſtances are retained long in the body, by their viſcidity. Dr. Ruſſel, in his Natural Hiſtory of Aleppo, relates, that in thoſe ſeaſons when oil abounds, the inhabitants by indulgence in it, are diſpoſed to fever, and affected with infarctions of the lungs; maladies which indicate both retention and obſtruction. Milk has been ſuſpected, by ſome, of producing ſimilar effects, though in a ſlighter degree; and the free uſe of it has been, on this account, forbidden to aſthmatics. From my own perſonal experience I ſhould preſume, that it is commonly much longer in paſſing by the kidneys, than other liquids; and analogy would lead us to the ſame concluſion, concerning its influence on perſpiration.

Gum arabic might be a good ſubſtitute for ſalep, in the compoſition, which I have recommended. And as it will give ſuch firmneſs to the maſs, as to require manducation, the ſaliva, by this means ſeparated and carried into the ſtomach, would further contribute to aſſuage the ſenſations both of hunger and of thirſt. We are informed by a traveller of veracity, that the Abyſſinians take an annual journey to Cairo, to ſell the products of their country; and that, as they paſs over vaſt deſerts, the duration of their rout is no leſs uncertain than a voyage at ſea. In the year 1750, the caravan had conſumed

ſumed all their proviſions, and were under the neceſſity of ſearching amongſt their merchandize, for ſomething wherewith to ſupport life, under that extremity. They found a ſufficient ſtock of gum arabic; and more than a thouſand perſons ſubſiſted upon it ſolely, for the ſpace of two months. The caravan arrived in ſafety at Cairo, without having ſuſtained any extraordinary loſſes, either by hunger or diſeaſe *(r)*. This gum, combined with ſugar and the whites of eggs, has been lately extolled in France, as a remedy for catarrhal defluxions. I have ſeen cakes made of theſe ingredients, and think they might very well be applied to the purpoſe of obviating hunger. They are not periſhable in the hotteſt climates, may be carried about the perſon with convenience, and though very tough, are pleaſant to the taſte. In the formula by which they are made, the proportion of ſugar is too large, and that of gum arabic too ſmall, if the maſs be intended to aſſuage the cravings of appetite. According to my information, the receipt is as follows. Take of fine ſugar four ounces, and of gum arabic one ounce: Levigate them well together, and add half an ounce of roſe water, and of the whites of eggs a ſufficient quantity.

(r) Haſſelquiſt's Voyages in the Levant, p. 298.

In our attempts to recover thoſe who have ſuffered under the calamities of famine, great circumſpection is required. Warmth, cordials, and food are the means to be employed; and it is evident that theſe may prove too powerful in their operation, if not adminiſtered with caution and judgment. For the body, by long faſting, is reduced to a ſtate of more than infantile debility; the minuter veſſels of the brain, and of the other organs, collapſe for want of fluids to diſtend them; the ſtomach and inteſtines ſhrink in their capacity; and the heart languidly vibrates, having ſcarcely ſufficient energy to propel the ſcanty current of blood. Under ſuch circumſtances, the treatment of Travis was proper, with reſpect to the application of heat, by placing, on each ſide, a healthy man in contact with him. *Pediluvia* or fomentations might, alſo, have been uſed with advantage. The temperature of theſe ſhould be lower than that of the human body, and gradually increaſed, according to the effects of their ſtimulus. New milk, weak broth, or water gruel ought to be employed both for the one and the other, as nutriment may be conveyed into the ſyſtem, this way, by paſſages, probably the moſt pervious in a ſtate of faſting, if not too long protracted. "A lad at New-market, a few years ago, hav-" "ing been almoſt ſtarved, in order that he might" "be

" be reduced to a proper weight, for riding a " match, was weighed at nine o'clock in the " morning, and again at ten; and he was found " to have gained near thirty ounces in weight, " in the courſe of an hour, though he had only " drank half a glaſs of wine in the interval. The " wine probably ſtimulated the action of the " nervous ſyſtem, and incited nature, exhauſted " by abſtinence, to open the abſorbent pores of " the whole body, in order to ſuck in ſome " nouriſhment from the air *(s)*." But no ſuch abſorption, as this, can be expected, in a ſtate of extreme weakneſs and emaciation, gradually induced; becauſe the lymphatics muſt partake of the general want of tone and energy. And notwithſtanding the ſalutary effects of wine, in the caſe of the jockey, who, it is likely, had been reduced by ſweating as well as by abſtinence, ſuch a ſtimulant might prove dangerous, and even fatal to one in the ſituation of Travis. I ſhould, therefore, adviſe the exhibition of cordials in very ſmall doſes, and, at firſt, conſiderably diluted. Slender wine whey will perhaps beſt anſwer this purpoſe; and afford, at the ſame time, an eaſy and pleaſant nouriſhment. When the ſtomach has been a little ſtrengthened, an egg may be mixed with the whey, or admini-

(s) Biſhop Watſon's Chemical Eſſays, vol. III. p. 101.

ſtered

ſtered under ſome other agreeable form. The yolk of one was, to Cornaro, ſufficient for a meal. And the narrative of this noble Venetian, in whom a fever was excited by the addition of only two ounces of food to his daily allowance, ſhews, that the return to a full diet ſhould be conducted with great caution, and by very ſlow gradations.

Though, I fear, my commentary has been already extended to an undue length, yet I cannot cloſe it, without ſoliciting the attention of the Society, to one additional circumſtance, in the caſe of Travis, peculiarly intereſting in its conſequences; viz. the eaſe with which he breathed, for a conſiderable ſpace of time, air too impure for candles to burn in, and which the men, who went in ſearch of him, durſt not venture to inſpire. As he had been long aſthmatic, we may reaſonably conclude, from his ſuffering ſo little, that the commonly received opinion of the *ſuffocating* nature of the *mephitis* or choke-damp, that it deſtroys the elaſticity of the air, and occaſions a collapſion of the lungs, is without foundation, notwithſtanding all the reſpectable authorities, which may be advanced in ſupport of it. Indeed, from the *phænomena* which attend the extinction of life, in thoſe to whom ſuch vapours have proved mortal, it is evident, that the poiſon acts chiefly on the nervous ſyſ-

tem.

tem. The vital principle ſeems to be arreſted, and almoſt inſtantaneouſly deſtroyed; ſometimes even without a ſtruggle, and, poſſibly, without any antecedent pain. Pliny the elder was found, after the fatal eruption of Mount Veſuvius, exactly in the ſame poſture in which he fell, with the appearance of one aſleep, rather than dead: *Habitus corporis quieſcenti quam defuncto ſimilior (t).* Some perſons killed by foul air in a cellar at Paris, were ſtiff as ſtatues, with their eyes open, and in the poſture of digging *(u)*. M. Beaumè relates the hiſtory of a man, who was recovered from apparent death, produced by a ſimilar cauſe, and who aſſerted, that he had felt neither pain nor oppreſſion; but that at the point of time when he was loſing his ſenſes, he experienced a delightful kind of delirium *(x)*. If, under ſuch circumſtances, this perſon could be ſufficiently collected to notice his feelings, the teſtimony is deciſive, that *oppreſſion* was not one of them; and conſequently, that he could not ſuffer from *ſuffocation*. And the account receives ſome confirmation from what Dr. Heberden ſays, in his lectures on poiſons, that he had ſeen an inſtance, in which the fumes of charcoal brought on the ſame delirium,

(t) Plinii Epiſt. XVI. lib. VI.

(u) Bomare Dict. d'Hiſtoire Naturelle.

(x) Roſier. Obſervations de la Phyſique. Jan. 1, 1774.

delirium, which hen-bane, and other intoxicating vegetables produce. Abbé Fontana breathed a certain portion of inflammable air, not only without inconvenience, but with unusual pleasure. He had a facility in dilating the breast, and never felt an equally agreeable sensation, even when he inhaled the purest dephlogisticated air. But he suffered greatly from this gratification, in a subsequent experiment: For, having filled a bladder with about three hundred and fifty cubic inches of inflammable air, he began to breathe it boldly, after discharging the atmospheric air, contained in his lungs, by a violent expiration. The first inspiration produced a great oppression: Towards the middle of the second, he was observed to become very pale, and objects appeared confused to his eyes: Nevertheless, he made a third inspiration. His strength now failed, he lost his sight entirely, fell upon his knees, and soon afterwards upon the floor. His respiration continued to be effected with difficulty and pain, as if he had a weight upon his breast; and he did not perfectly recover before the succeeding day *(y)*.

In this instance, some degree of palsy was probably induced, in the nerves of the lungs, by the sudden action of concentrated inflammable air,

(y) Philosoph. Transf. vol. LXIX. p. 346.

conveyed

conveyed into the vesicles, forcibly emptied of atmospheric air. For in ordinary respiration, about thirty five cubic inches of air are inhaled and exhaled; but in a violent expiration, the air discharged may amount to sixty cubic inches (z). In the case of Travis, it will be remembered, that the air was sufficiently salubrious, when he went down into the coal pit; that by stagnation it became gradually noxious; and that his nervous system must therefore have been progressively habituated to its influence. This is conformable to the observations of my friend Dr. Priestley, who discovered, that if a mouse can bear the first shock of being put into a vessel, filled with artificial gas, or if the gas be increased by degrees, it will live, a considerable time, in a situation which would prove instantly fatal to other mice. And he frequently noticed, that when a number of mice had been confined, in a given quantity of infected air, a fresh mouse introduced amongst them, has presently died in convulsions.

The same ingenious philosopher seems to have ascertained, that respiration is a phlogistic process; that it is the office of the lungs to carry off the putrid *effluvium*, or to discharge the phlogiston, introduced into the system with the

(z) Id. p. 349.

aliment,

aliment, and become effete; and that the air we breathe acts, on this occasion, as a *menstruum:* We are also assured, by an able chemist, that the quantity of air, phlogisticated by a man in a minute, is equal to that, which is phlogisticated by a candle, in the same space of time *(a)*. Hence it might be presumed, that like supplies of atmospheric air are essential to respiration and combustion. But the experience of Travis proves the fact to be otherwise *(b)*. And though miners generally try the salubrity of the subterraneous air, by the test of a lighted candle, yet we are informed by Mr. Keir, that he has seen them working in the shaft of a coal pit, several yards below that part where the candle was extinguished. Indeed it was observed by Mr. Boyle, and has since been confirmed by Dr. Priestley, that an animal will live nearly, if not quite, as long in air, in which candles have burned out, as in common air. There must be some power, therefore, it should seem, in the living œconomy, to free the body from redundant phlogiston, by other emunctories than the lungs: or a small portion of atmospheric air may suffice,

(a) See Crawford on Animal Heat, p. 80.

(b) DR. PRIESTLEY informs me, that he has lately bestowed particular attention on a kind of air, in which a candle burns, but in which a mouse will not live.

for this purpoſe, in extraordinary emergencies, and for a ſhort period of time. This accommodating faculty, if I may ſo expreſs it, is evidenced in various other inſtances, and particularly in one, no leſs remarkable than that, of which we are now treating: I mean, the equality of temperature, which the body retains, in great extremes of heat and cold. A Ruſſian Boor, in the winter ſeaſon, daily experiences all theſe varieties of air, of heat, and of cold, without inconvenience. When labouring out of doors, he is expoſed to the intenſity of froſt and ſnow: When he retires in the evening, to his hut, which conſiſts only of one cloſe apartment, never ventilated during ſix months, he feeds upon ſalted fiſh or fleſh, and afterwards repoſes on a greaſy mattreſs, placed over an oven, in which billets of wood are burned. In this ſituation he is literally ſtewed, with his whole family, who live in a conſtant ſteam, not offenſive to themſelves, but ſo groſs and noiſome, as to be ſcarcely ſupportable by a ſtranger *(c)*. The atmoſphere of a crowded town muſt, in many reſpects, reſemble the foul air of a Ruſſian cottage; yet thouſands enjoy in it a tolerable ſhare of health.

(c) See Phil. Tranſ. vol. LXVIII. p. 622.

IT

It has been found, by experiment, that the fumes emitted by almoft every fpecies of burning fuel, are fatal to animals, when applied in a fufficiently concentrated ftate. I have computed, that three hundred tons of coal are every day confumed, in the winter feafon, at Manchefter. The factitious *gas*, generated by its combuftion, muft amount at leaft to one third of this quantity; it is probable that the fmoke, proceeding from it, conftitutes another third part; and both together are capable of occupying a fpace of very wide extent. If it were not for the difperfion of thefe vapours by wind, the precipitation of them by rain, and the influence of other caufes, which reftore falubrity to the air, refpiration could not be carried on, in fuch circumftances. And we may obferve that frofty weather, which is generally ferene and without wind, always proves extremely oppreffive, and fometimes even fatal to afthmatic patients, in great cities. Indeed the rate of human mortality bears a pretty near proportion to their magnitude and population: And I have fhewn, in another Effay, that there is an aftonifhing difference between the expectation of life in Manchefter, and the country immediately furrounding it, although the inhabitants of both are fubject to the fame viciffitudes of weather, carry on the fame manufactures, are fupplied with provisions from the same market, and, by their free intercourse, are almost equally liable to attacks of small-pox, fevers, and other epidemics.

It is evident, therefore, that habit, however it may abate, cannot entirely counteract the baneful operation of bad air. And those will feel its pernicious effects most strongly, in every situation, whose nervous systems are endued with more than ordinary sensibility. Such persons I would caution not to indulge their curiosity in the inspection of unwholesome manufactures, nor in visiting mines, caverns, stoves, hospitals, or prisons. Several gentlemen, in this assembly, will recollect that the late Dr. Brown suffered, in a very acute degree, by accompanying two foreigners of distinction into the Duke of Bridgewater's works, at Worsley. It happened they were the first, who entered the tunnel, on that day. The candles, which they carried with them, were observed to burn very dimly; but neither the passengers nor the boatmen experienced any difficulty in respiration. After remaining in the coal pits a considerable time, they proceeded to Warrington; where Dr. Brown was attacked with violent pains, which shifted suddenly from one part of his body to another. Small purple spots overspread his skin; his throat became so tumefied as to render swallowing difficult; and great prostration of strength, with

with a low fever enſued. The Doctor was ſubject to the anomalous gout, had once a paralytic complaint of long continuance, and hence we may conclude that his nervous ſyſtem was endued with peculiar irritability. He was not, however, the ſole ſufferer; for one of the foreigners was affected with ſimilar *petechiæ*, but attended with little pain or diſorder.

LAST year a general alarm was ſpread, in this neighbourhood, concerning the danger, ariſing from the noiſome effluvia of certain cotton works, to all employed, or who had communication with thoſe employed in them. But the good ſenſe and humanity of the proprietors, aided by the authority and patriotic exertions of our magiſtrates, have quieted theſe apprehenſions, by removing, in no inconſiderable degree, the cauſes from which they originated *(f)*. And, I truſt, the factories are now tolerably well ventilated, ſupplied with purer oil, and kept in a ſtate of greater cleanlineſs. Still, however, the delicate and valetudinary incur a riſk in viſiting them. For foul air, though it contain not any contagious particles, may yet poſſeſs a virulence, that is capable, in particular habits, of producing

(f) SEE a copy of the paper, printed and diſtributed, by order of the magiſtrates, at the cloſe of this Eſſay; which will ſhew the meaſures taken on the intereſting occaſion referred to.

ducing fever. Like certain poiſons, it effects an inſtantaneous change in the nervous ſyſtem, by which the organs of ſecretion are diſturbed, and the ſecretions themſelves corrupted. The common precautions, therefore, ought not to be neglected by thoſe who expoſe themſelves to the influence of ſuch vapours. The valetudinary, eſpecially, ſhould not enter the works with an empty ſtomach, ſhould previouſly fortify themſelves by a glaſs or two of wine, and counteract the ſedative operation of the putrid miaſms by the ſtimulus of hartſhorn, *eau de luce*, or camphorated vinegar, applied to the noſe. But theſe volatile ſubſtances are to be ſuffered, as much as poſſible, to riſe ſpontaneouſly, and not to be drawn forcibly into the noſtrils: For by ſuch inhalation the noxious atoms, floating in the air, will be conveyed to the olfactory nerves, with additional energy; and, being lodged in the ſchneiderian membrane, they may exert their baneful powers, when the action of the antidote ſhall ceaſe. To this cauſe is to be aſcribed that permanency of offenſive ſmells, which makes us ſenſible to their impreſſion, ſome time after our removal from their ſource. And, when this impreſſion is no longer perceived, in the ordinary courſe of reſpiration, it may often be renewed by that effort which we denominate ſnuffing. In this way, I apprehend, and

and not ſolely from abſorption, the fact is to be explained which Mr. Howard has related, that his phial of vinegar, after uſing it in a few priſons, became intolerably diſagreeable to him. When a malignant contagion prevails in hoſpitals, gaols, or pariſh work-houſes, it is to be feared that the preventives, I have recommended, will afford no adequate ſecurity. They may, however, be of ſome avail; and it would ſurely be raſhneſs and preſumption to neglect them altogether. But firmer grounds of confidence may reaſonably influence the minds of thoſe, who are led by official or profeſſional duty to incur ſuch dangers. "I have been frequently "aſked," ſays the humane writer whom I have juſt quoted, and with whoſe words I ſhall now cloſe this commentary, "what precautions I "uſe to preſerve myſelf from infection, in the "priſons and hoſpitals which I viſit. I here "anſwer, that next to the free goodneſs and "mercy of the Author of my being, temperance "and cleanlineſs are my preſervatives. Truſting "in *Divine Providence*, and believing myſelf in "the way of my *duty*, I viſit the moſt noxious "cells; and, while thus employed, *I fear no* "*evil.*"

A COPY of the PAPER printed and diſtributed by Order of the MAGISTRATES of the County Palatine of LANCASTER, at the MICHAELMAS SESSIONS, 1784.

COUNTY OF LANCASTER.

A REPRESENTATION, of a very alarming nature, having been made by Lord Grey de Wilton, and a great number of the moſt reſpectable inhabitants of the townſhip and neighbourhood of Radcliffe, in this county, to the GENTLEMEN to whom the following letter is directed, of a malignant fever, which was ſuppoſed to have originated in the cotton works there; they took the liberty of deſiring Dr. Percival, and the other Medical Gentlemen of Mancheſter, to take upon themſelves, the trouble of making ſuch inquiries, as they ſhould think neceſſary, in order to aſcertain the cauſes to which it was owing; and the moſt proper methods to be uſed, to prevent the further ſpreading of the contagion. Much to the credit of the phyſicians, they undertook the taſk with the greateſt alacrity; went over to the infected place themſelves; and the following report was the conſequence.

To SAMUEL CLOWES, jun.
THOMAS B. BAYLEY,
DORNING RASBOTHAM,
M. BENTLEY, } Eſquires.

His Majeſty's Juſtices of the Peace, for the County Palatine of Lancaſter.

GENTLEMEN,

GENTLEMEN,

WE have taken into the moſt deliberate conſideration, your very humane and judicious requiſition; and we ſhall now lay before you the reſult of our inquiries, concerning thoſe intereſting objects, which you have propoſed to our inveſtigation. We have fully ſatisfied ourſelves, either from actual obſervation, or authentic teſtimony, that a low, putrid fever, of a contagious nature, has prevailed many months in the cotton mills, and amongſt the poor, in the townſhip of Radcliffe. We cannot, however, aſcertain, whether this fever originated in thoſe works, or was imported into Radcliffe from ſome other parts of the county. But though this point remain doubtful, we are decided in our opinion—That the diſorder has been ſupported, diffuſed, and aggravated, by the ready communication of contagion to numbers crowded together; by the acceſſion to its virulence from putrid effluvia; and by the injury done to young perſons through confinement, and too long continued labour; to which ſeveral evils the cotton mills have given occaſion.

THESE evils, we truſt, are not without remedy; and from the benevolent attention, which the proprietors of the Radcliffe works have ſhewn to the ſick and infirm under their charge, we may reaſonably preſume to hope, they will be induced to adopt the following practicable regulations, from motives of policy, humanity, and juſtice, as well as from the reſpect, which is due to your authority.

I. ALL the caſements of the windows, and the three large weſtern doors of the cotton mills, ſhould be left open every night: The ſame regulation ſhould take place, during the receſs from work, at noon; and as many caſements ſhould be kept open, in the hours of labour, as may be compatible with carrying on the operations of the machinery.

II. THE

II. The cafements are too fmall; being in dimenfion, only about one fixth part of the window. They are likewife placed high, and parallel to each other—a pofition obvioufly unfavourable to complete ventilation: For the inlet of the air ought to be lower than the outlet.

III. Several fire-places, with open chimneys, fhould be erected, at proper diftances, in each work room. The ftoves, now employed, afford no fufficient paffage for the offenfive vapours generated in the rooms; and increafe the contamination of the air, by the effluvia which they emit. Turf would be the cheapeft, and alfo a very falutary fuel; for it confifts, chiefly, of the roots of vegetables; and yields, in burning, a ftrong, penetrating, and pungent fmoke, which is likely to prove as good an antidote to contagion, as that of wood is found to be, from long experience.

IV. The rooms fhould be daily fwept, and the floors wafhed, at leaft once every week, with ftrong lime-water, or with water impregnated with the fpirit of vitriol, or the acid of tar. The walls and cielings may be fcraped and white-wafhed, at firft, every month, and afterwards, twice or thrice yearly. Lime frefh burnt, and as foon as it is flaked, muft be ufed for this purpofe, and the wafh laid on whilft it is hot.

V. During the prevalence of the prefent fever, the apartments fhould be fumigated weekly with tobacco. Brimftone would, perhaps, be more powerful, but, in burning, it yields an acid, which might be iujurious to the cotton.

VI. Great attention ought to be paid to the privies. They fhould be wafhed daily; and ventilated in fuch a manner, that the fmell arifing from them fhall not be perceptible in the work rooms.

VII. The

VII. The rancid oil, which is employed in the machinery, is a copious ſource of putrid effluvia. We apprehend, that a purer oil would be much leſs unwholeſome, and that the additional expence of it would be fully compenſated, by its ſuperior power in diminiſhing friction.

VIII. A strict obſervance of cleanlineſs ſhould be enjoined on all who work in the mills, as an efficacious mean of preventing contagion, and of preſerving health. It may alſo be adviſable to bathe the children occaſionally. The apparel of thoſe who are infected with the preſent fever, ſhould be well fumigated, before it is again worn. And the linen, &c. of the ſick, ſhould firſt be waſhed in *cold* water, leſt the ſteams ariſing from heat communicate the diſtemper to the perſons engaged in that operation. Crofter's lye, when it can be procured, is preferable to water. The bodies of thoſe who die of the fever, ſhould be cloſely wrapped in pitched cloth; and interred as ſoon as propriety or decency will permit. Smoking tobacco will be an uſeful preſervative to the ſuperintendants of the works, and to others expoſed to infection, who can practiſe it with convenience.

IX. We earneſtly recommend a longer receſs from labour at noon, and a more early diſmiſſion from it in the evening, to all who work in the cotton mills. But we deem this indulgence eſſential to the preſent health, and future capacity for labour, of thoſe who are under the age of fourteen. For the active recreations of childhood and youth are neceſſary to the growth, the vigour, and the right conformation of the human body. And we cannot excuſe ourſelves, on the preſent occaſion, from ſuggeſting to you, who are the guardians of the public weal, this further very important conſideration, that the riſing generation ſhould not be debarred from all opportunities of inſtruction,

inſtruction, at the only ſeaſon of life, in which they can be properly improved.

We have the honour to be, with the higheſt reſpect,

GENTLEMEN, your moſt faithful,

and obedient humble ſervants,

THOMAS PERCIVAL, M.D.
JOHN COWLING, M.D.
ALEXANDER EASON, M.D.
EDWOOD CHORLEY, M.D.

MANCHESTER,
October 8, 1784.

P. S. OUR reſpectable colleagues, Dr. Mainwaring and Dr. Mitchell, are abſent from Mancheſter at this time.

MANCHESTER MICHAELMAS SESSIONS, 1784.

THE magiſtrates of this county, aſſembled in their general quarter ſeſſions at Mancheſter, impreſſed with the obligations they are under, have directed the clerk of the peace to give their public thanks to Dr. Percival, Dr. Cowling, Dr. Eaſon, and Dr. Chorley; and to take care that their letter ſhall be printed and diſtributed, ſo that every part of the community may receive the benefit of their ſalutary admonitions, a ſtrict attention to which is moſt earneſtly recommended by the court. By order of the court,

JAMES TAYLOR,
Deputy-clerk of the peace for the county of Lancaſter.

ESSAY

ESSAY VI.

A PHYSICAL INQUIRY INTO THE POWERS AND OPERATION OF MEDICINES:

Addreſſed to the LITERARY and PHILOSOPHICAL SOCIETY, of MANCHESTER (a).

MEDICINES are the inſtruments employed for the preſervation of health, or the cure of diſeaſes: It muſt therefore, be an object of intereſting ſpeculation to the philoſopher, and of practical importance to the phyſician, to inveſtigate the *rationale* of their action on the human body. But there is no branch of the healing art which is in itſelf more intricate and obſcure; nor any one that has undergone ſo many doctrinal viciſſitudes. It would treſpaſs too much

(a) INSERTED in the third volume of the Memoirs of the Literary and Philoſophical Society.

much on the time allotted for ſuch diſcuſſions, in this ſociety, to enumerate the multifarious hypotheſes, which have been ſupported by the ſucceſſive ſectaries in phyſic, ſince the days of Hippocrates. On many of theſe I have animadverted in an Eſſay, publiſhed near twenty years ago *(b)*. And I ſhall now only requeſt your candid attention to a few obſervations, on the opinions which are beginning to prevail in our ſchools; and your permiſſion to offer ſome hints towards the extenſion of our views, and the methodizing of our experience, relative to this curious and philoſophical ſubject.

ANATOMY has revealed the exquiſite ſtructure of our corporeal frame; and phyſiology has taught us that, in its animated ſtate, the organs of which it is compoſed are reciprocally connected with, and delicately adjuſted to each other. The nerves, though productions of the brain, apparently ſimilar, are yet endued with powers and ſenſibilities widely diverſified. This is evident to the moſt ſuperficial obſerver, in the ſeveral SENSES: And the nerves of every other part of the body have probably, in like manner, their appropriate faculties; all adapted to diſtinct offices, but tending to one common end, the health, ſupport, and perfection of the animal

(b) Vol. I. Eſſay I.

nature. The minuteſt agent, therefore, may excite a movement capable of being propagated to any part of the ſyſtem, or even through the whole of it, by a ſympathetic energy independent and far beyond the power of the primary inſtrument of motion. From theſe premiſes it is now generally inferred, agreeably to the ſimplicity which ſubſiſts in all the operations of nature, "that a medicine is only the *cauſe of a cauſe*, "according to the phraſe of the logicians; that "its proper action is confined to the nerves or "fibres to which it is immediately applied; that "when received into the ſtomach, after the firſt "impreſſion on the very ſenſible coats of that "organ, the nature of it is gradually changed, "by the ſolvent powers of the gaſtric juices; "and that if incapable of being digeſted into a "mild and nutritious chyle, it is carried through "the inteſtinal canal, and ejected as uſeleſs and "noxious to the body."

Error may be built on the baſis of acknowledged, if only partial, truth; and is then moſt ſpecious in its form, and moſt authoritative in its influence on the underſtanding. But the impoſition ceaſes when we extend our views. And I ſhall endeavour to ſhew, that the operation of medicines is to be meaſured by a more enlarged ſcale than the foregoing hypotheſis, or any

any other which now occurs to my recollection, applies to it.

I. Medicines may act on the human body by an immediate and peculiar impression on the stomach and bowels, either in their proper form; in a state of decomposition; or by new powers acquired from combination, or a change in the arrangement of their parts. The ſympathy of the ſtomach with the whole animated ſyſtem is ſo obvious to our daily experience, that it cannot require much illuſtration.. After faſting and fatigue, we feel that a moderate quantity of wine inſtantly exhilarates the ſpirits, and gives energy to all the muſcular fibres of the body. It has been known even to produce a ſudden and large augmentation of weight, after much depletion, by rouſing the abſorbent ſyſtem to vigorous action. Such power is peculiar to living mechaniſm; and is properly denominated, by phyſicians, the *vis medicatrix naturæ.* But apparent as is the ſympathy of the ſtomach, the laws, by which it is governed, are very inſufficiently underſtood: And we have hitherto learned only from a looſe induction of facts, that the nerves of this delicate organ ſeem to be endued with diverſified ſenſibilities; that impreſſions, made by the ſame or different ſubſtances, have their appropriate influence on different

different and diſtant parts; and that the ſtomach itſelf undergoes frequent variations in its ſtates of irritability. A few grains of blue vitriol, taken internally, excite inſtantly the moſt violent contractions of the abdominal, and other muſcles concerned in vomiting. A doſe of *ipecacuanha*, as ſoon as it produces nauſea, abates both the force and velocity of the heart, in its vital motion; and affects the whole ſeries of blood veſſels, from their origin to their minuteſt ramifications; as is evident by the paleneſs of the ſkin, under ſuch circumſtances, and by the efficacy of emetics in ſtopping hæmorrhages. The head, when diſordered with vertigo, ſometimes derives ſudden relief from a tea ſpoonful or two of æther, adminiſtered in a glaſs of water. And I have known an inceſſant cough to attack the lungs, in conſequence of the ſtimulus of a pin, which had been unwarily ſwallowed. Of the action of medicines on the ſtomach, under decompoſition or recompoſition, we have an example, familiar to every one, in magneſia. For this abſorbent earth by neutralizing the acid in the *primæ viæ*, acquires a purgative quality, and at the ſame time yields a gas of great ſalubrity, as an anti emetic, tonic, and antiſeptic.

II. Medicines may pass into the course of circulation, in one or other of the states

ABOVE DESCRIBED; AND, BEING CONVEYED TO DIFFERENT AND DISTANT PARTS, MAY EXERT CERTAIN APPROPRIATE ENERGIES. Chemiſtry furniſhes numberleſs caſes wherein ſubſtances undergo changes, and put on new forms more remarkable than can be effected by the digeſtion of the ſtomach, retaining ſtill the *materia prima*, and being capable of reſuming the original arrangement of their particles, and conſequently their original qualities. Now, a body altered in its texture, by the digeſtive organs, and carried into the ſyſtem with the aliment, may by ſuch alteration acquire ſpecific powers on particular ſound or diſeaſed parts. Thus, if we ſuppoſe cantharides to be changed in form and texture, when mixed with the chyle, the lymph, or blood, yet in that form and texture they may be peculiarly adapted to excite ſtrangury in the urinary paſſages. Or, we may conceive that this new modification of their corpuſcles may again be altered, and their original compoſition reſtored by a ſubſequent chemical change in the kidneys; an event not more ſingular than the ſeparation of urine from the blood, than the revival of a metal, or the precipitation of a ſolvend from its menſtruum by elective attraction. The urinary excretion ſeems to be deſigned by nature to carry off the recrementitious parts of the circulating fluids. And it clearly ſhews what compoſitions,

compoſitions, and decompoſitions take place in the body. For it varies almoſt every hour, both in the ſtate of health and of diſeaſe; and the lateritious, pinky, mucous, and other appearances it exhibits, are the reſult of chemical changes, either in itſelf, or in the fluids from which it is derived.

THE ſenſible qualities of any body are no certain criteria of its medicinal action. Peruvian bark owes not its efficacy to bitterneſs; for ſtronger bitters are not poſſeſſed of its febrifuge powers. Antimony, though inſipid, is violent in its operation on the nerves of the ſtomach: And yet, if applied to the eye, an organ endued with equal ſenſibility, it is entirely inert. To what property in opium, capable of affecting the external ſenſes, are we to aſcribe its narcotic powers? Or is there, in the grateful taſte of *ſaccharum ſaturni*, any indication of a deadly poiſon? But the inſtances are numberleſs, which may be adduced to prove the uncertainty of reaſoning otherwiſe than from obſervation, concerning the action of medicines, and the peculiar ſenſibility of different parts of our ſyſtem to their impreſſion. Following, therefore, experience as our guide, let us notice ſuch facts as may elucidate the ſubject before us. It is well known that madder root carries its tinging quality to the bones, affecting neither the ſkin, the muſcles, the ligaments, nor fat. Digeſtion conſequently leaves this tinging quality unchanged; or perhaps it is again recovered, when arrived at the bones, by ſome new arrangement of parts produced by the chemiſtry of nature *(c)*. Extract of logwood, taken internally, ſometimes gives a bloody hue to the urine. But the aſtringency of it does not, according to my trials, accompany its colouring matter *(d)*. I recollect no inſtance wherein the milk either of a nurſe, or of an animal, was tinged with madder or logwood. This affords ſome preſumption that the pigment does not ſubſiſt, in its proper form, in the blood; but that it is recovered by a ſubſequent

(c) THE bones of the Canada Porcupine, during winter, are of a greeniſh yellow, owing, as is ſuppoſed, to the bark of the pine on which the animal feeds in that ſeaſon of the year. See Pennant's Arctic Zoology, p. 110. N°. 42.

(d) IT is ſaid the fruit of the Nopal, or Indian fig, on which the cochineal is propagated, tinges the urine of thoſe who eat it, with a deep blood colour. The leaves of this ſhrub are of a permanent and lively green; and it is remarkable that their juices are converted, by the concoctive organs of the inſect which feeds on them, into a dye exactly ſimilar to that produced by the powers of vegetation in the pulp of the fruit. Cartheuſer obtained from the cochineal a moderately *aſtringent* ſpirituous extract, amounting, in weight, nearly to three fourths of the ſubſtance from which it was prepared. Theſe facts exhibit a ſtriking analogy between digeſtion and vegetation, as the products appear to be the ſame both in colour and quality.

change,

change, in the diſpoſition of its conſtituent particles. And if one ſubſtance ſtain the bones, by being carried into contact with them, another may, in a way analogous, produce in them fragility or diſſolution. In the diſeaſe termed by the French *ergot*, and which, with apparent reaſon, is aſcribed to the uſe of a ſpecies of unſound corn, the bones loſe the earthy matter that enters into their texture, and become ſoft and eaſy to be broken. This effect is gradual, and probably ariſes from ſome unknown quality of the corn, which is either not ſubdued by digeſtion, or reſumed in the juices that circulate through the oſſeous veſſels. A change in the proceſs of vegetation may communicate a diſſolvent power to an eſculent ſeed. Muſtard acquires it by its natural growth, and is capable of rendering even ivory itſelf ſoft and fragile. How far it would produce ſuch an effect on the bones of a living body, if uſed as the chief article of diet, we have no experience on which to ground any ſatisfactory concluſion. The peaſantry, in the mountainous parts of this county, who live on oat meal, are peculiarly liable to cutaneous eruptions. Theſe have ſometimes been aſcribed to obſtructed perſpiration. But ſuch obſtruction is itſelf only a concomitant effect of ſome quality in the oat meal, injurious to the ſkin.

Sulphur, whether externally or internally uſed, produces a cure in the itch. In each way, therefore, we may preſume its operation to be ſimilar. But when taken into the ſtomach, there can be no doubt that it undergoes a change in the modification of its parts, and that it does not circulate through the blood veſſels either in the form, or with the properties of ſulphur. Yet when conveyed to the ſurface of the body, it appears evidently to recover its original powers, communicating its peculiar odour to the perſpiration, tinging ſilver, and curing cutaneous defœdations *(e)*. The ſame holds true of the vitriolic acid, when adminiſtered in large doſes. It ſeems to acquire phlogiſton in the animal body, and to paſs off by the pores, as hepatic air, or as volatilized ſulphur. Even when given to nurſes, it proves an effectual remedy for the itch, both in them, and the children whom they ſuckle.

(e) Bishop Watson, in his Chemical Eſſays, warns thoſe who uſe coſmetic lotions containing ceruſſe, to forbear from them at Harrowgate, Moffat, or other places where they drink ſulphurated waters, "leſt they ſhould be in "the ſtate of the unlucky fair one, whoſe face, neck, and "arms were ſuddenly deſpoiled of all their beauties, and "changed quite black." Vol. III. p. 365. And his Lordſhip informs me, that there is an inſtance mentioned in the German Ephemerides, of a perſon who had taken ſo much elixir of vitriol, that his keys were ruſted in his pocket, by the tranſudation of the acid through his ſkin.

ſuckle. Mercury, combined with ſulphur into an æthiops, has been generally regarded as inert. But inſtances have occurred, in which, under this form, though accurately prepared, it has produced ſalivation; an evident proof of a chemical change in the æthiops, by which the mercury was reſtored to its priſtine powers. Indeed the ſame reaſoning may be applied to the ſpecific action of mercury on the ſalival glands, in whatever mode it be adminiſtered *(f)*. A ptyaliſm is ſometimes produced by antimony. Dr. James aſſured my friend Sir George Baker, that he knew ſix inſtances of it, occaſioned by his fever powder, although he had left mercury out of its compoſition long before they occurred. But the patients, thus affected, had neither their teeth looſened, nor their breath made offenſive.

Most perſons have experienced the effects of aſparagus on the urine *(g)*. This takes place

(f) We have the concurrent teſtimony of many authors, that mercury has been found, reſtored to its original form, in the carious bones of their patients. Vid. Joan. Farnel. cap. 7. Gabriel. Fallop. cap. 78. Joan Languem, lib. I. epiſt. XLIII. Alex. Petrom. cap. 1. lib. VI. &c. &c.

(g) Cabbage, eſpecially that of the winter's growth, impregnates water with a diſagreeable ſmell, ſomewhat ſimilar to that which is communicated by aſparagus. Yet, I believe, cabbage is never known to taint the urine; perhaps from its having no chemical affinity with it.

 very

very ſpeedily and ſtrongly too, though a ſmall quantity only has been eaten. The ſmell is much more diſagreeable than that of aſparagus itſelf. And as the odorous particles conveyed to the kidneys muſt be greatly diluted in their paſſage (even on the ſuppoſition of the retrograde motion of the lymphatics, which does not ſeem probable in a caſe ſo invariable and uniform) I ſhould conceive that a new combination of particles takes place in the urinary organs; and that the odorous part of the ſecretion differs in its form and quality, both from what ſubſiſted in the chyle and in the blood.

THERE are certain medicines which, when ſwallowed, quickly manifeſt themſelves in the diſcharges, with ſome of their original qualities. Soap lyes, when taken in large quantities, render the urine alkaline and lithontriptic: And the ſame excretion becomes impregnated with fixed air, if mephitic water be drunk freely. A patient, whom I viſit at this time, has ſix grains of the Balſam of Tolu adminiſtered to him thrice every day; and his urine is ſtrongly ſcented, even by this ſmall quantity. Fuller aſſerts of the Balſam of Copaiba, *Urinam odore violaceo minime inficit; illam vero ſapore amaro imbuit.* Garlick affects the breath, though applied only around the wriſts. The milk of a nurſe is, likewiſe, eaſily tainted with it. A purgative given to one who ſuckles will ſometimes

produce

produce no operation on her bowels, if ſhe be coſtive, but a powerful one on the child at her breaſt.—But a ſtill more convincing proof that there may be a renovation of the original qualities of a body, after it has undergone the proceſs of digeſtion, and other ſubſequent changes, is deducible from theſe facts; that butter is often impregnated with the taſte and ſmell of certain vegetables, on which the cows have paſtured; that the milk of ſuch cows diſcovers no diſagreeable flavour; neither does the whey nor cheeſe prepared from it. Now, butter is formed, firſt by a ſpontaneous ſeparation of cream; and ſecondly by a fermentation of it, that is, by a two-fold and ſucceſſive new arrangement of its elementary parts. By theſe changes, the original offenſive materials in the food of the cow ſeem to reaſſume their proper form and nature.

After venæſection the ſerum of the blood has ſometimes appeared as white as milk, whilſt the craſſamentum retained its natural colour. This whiteneſs hath been ſhewn to ariſe from oleaginous particles (not unaſſimilated chyle) floating in the circulating fluids *(b)*; and may ſerve to explain a fact, recorded by a writer of good authority, on the natural hiſtory of Aleppo, that "in certain ſeaſons, when oil is plentifully "taken, the people become diſpoſed to fevers

(b) See Hewſon on the Blood, p. 146.

"and

"and infarctions of the lungs; which symptoms "wear off by retrenching this indulgence *(i)*." Some years ago cod-liver oil was annually dispensed, amongst the sick in our hospital, to the amount of fifty or sixty gallons. The taste and smell are extremely nauseous; and it leaves upon the palate a savour like that of putrid fish. This remedy is most salutary when it operates by perspiration; and the sweat of those to whom it is administered, always becomes strongly tainted with it. An oil of the same kind forms no inconsiderable part of the food of many northern nations; and it is said to penetrate and imbue the deepest recesses of the body *(k)*.

In the Philosophical Transactions for 1750, vol. I. part II. p. 295. Dr. Wright relates an experiment, to prove that chalybeates do not enter the blood. He forced a dog, which had fasted sixty-six hours, to swallow a pound of bread and milk, with which an ounce and a half of green vitriol were mixed. An hour afterwards he opened the dog, and collected from the thoracic duct near half an ounce of chyle, which assumed no change of colour when the

(i) See Russel's History of Aleppo.

(k) Oil was formerly administered in pregnancy, by Sir William Hamilton, and other experienced physicians, to promote easy delivery: But modern theory has superseded their observation and experience!

tincture

tincture of galls was dropped into it; though it acquired a deep purple from the ſame tincture, when one fourth of a grain of *ſal martis* had been diſſolved in it. This experiment is uſually deemed deciſive in ſupport of the theory, that chalybeates exert their operations ſolely on the ſtomach; and that the vigour they communicate to the ſyſtem ariſes, excluſively, from their tonic powers on the alimentary canal, and on the ſympathy of the ſtomach with various other parts of the body. I am not inclined to doubt either the tonic action or the ſympathy ſuppoſed; but I ſee not that they preclude the immediate agency of ſteel on remote parts of the human frame. For this remedy, in other forms capable of being introduced into the circulation, may exert conſiderable energy, as deobſtruent, ſtimulant, or aſtringent. And the experiment adduced only evinces, that it did not ſubſiſt in the chyle as a vitriol, qualified to ſtrike a black colour with galls. Neither does the calx of iron, nor the glaſs of iron poſſeſs this power: Yet, though changed, they are both capable of being reſtored to it. Perhaps, with equal reaſon, it might be preſumed, by one ignorant of chemiſtry, that *ſal martis* contains no iron, becauſe it is not acted upon by the load-ſtone.

With the foregoing obſervation of Dr. Wright, I ſhall contraſt thoſe made by the celebrated Dr.

Dr. Musgrave, which are also recorded in the annals of the Royal Society. " I injected," says he, " into the *jejunum* of a dog, that had, for a " day before, but little meat, about twelve " ounces of a solution of indigo in fountain " water, and after three hours, opening the dog " a second time, I observed several of the lac- " teals of a bluish colour, which, on stretching " the mesentery, did several times disappear, " but was most easily discerned when the me- " sentery lay loose, an argument that the bluish " liquor was not properly of the vessels, but of " the liquors contained in it. A few days after " this, repeating the experiment in another com- " pany, with the solution of stone blue in foun- " tain water, and on a dog that had been kept " fasting thirty-six hours, I saw several of the " lacteals become of a perfect blue colour within " very few minutes after the injection. For they " appeared before I could sew up the gut.

" About the beginning of March following, " having kept a spaniel fasting thirty-six hours, " and then syringing a pint of deep decoction of " stone blue with common water, into one of " the small guts; and after three hours, opening " the dog again, I saw many of the lacteals of a " deep blue colour, several of them were cut, " and afforded a blue liquor, some of the decoc- " tion running forth on the mesentery. After

" this

"this I examined the *ductus thoracicus*, (on which, "together with other veſſels near it, I had on "my return made a ligature) and ſaw the *receptaculum chyli*, and that *ductus* of a bluiſh colour; "not ſo blue indeed as the lacteals, from the "ſolution mixing, in or near the *receptaculum*, "with *lympha*; but much bluer than the *ductus* "uſed to be, or than the lymphatics under the "liver, with which I compared it, were *(l)*."

STONE BLUE is a preparation of cobalt, pot-aſh, and white lead; which, being converted into glaſs, is ground into a fine powder. And if ſuch a ſubſtance can pervade the lacteals, we may conclude that they are permeable to other bodies, beſides thoſe deſigned for nutrition, and capable of aſſimilation with the blood. This argument, from analogy, receives great additional force from the known fact that mercury, and various other active remedies, may be conveyed into the body through the abſorbents of the ſkin, a ſyſtem of veſſels, ſimilar to thoſe above-mentioned, in their ſtructure, uſes, and termination. In a caſe of *hydrocephalus internus*, on which I have lately been conſulted, a child under one year of age received, by ſucceſſive frictions, four ounces, ſix drachms, and two ſcruples of the *unguentum*

(l) SEE Philoſoph. Tranſ. abridged by Motte, chap. IV. part II. p. 76.

guentum

guentum cœruleum fortius, between the eighth of February and the ſeventh of April 1786. One ſcruple was adminiſtered each time; the operation took up more than half an hour; and the part, to which the ointment was applied, was always previouſly bathed with warm water; precautions which ſeemed to ſecure the full abſorption of the mercury *(m)*. I ſhould not omit to mention that the child recovered without any ſymptoms of ſalivation, and continues perfectly well. Indeed I have repeatedly obſerved, that very large quantities of the *unguentum cœruleum* may be uſed in infancy and childhood, without affecting the gums, notwithſtanding the prediſpoſition to a flux of ſaliva, at a period of life incident to dentition.

WHENCE is it that a medicine, ſo irritating as mercury, can be conveyed into the courſe of circulation, when even milk, or the mildeſt liquors, if transfuſed into the blood veſſels, have been found to produce convulſions and death? Is it that what paſſes by the lymphatics or lacteals

(m) Thirty-ſeven grains of calomel were given internally during this ſpace of time, at proper intervals, and in ſixteen doſes. The caſe referred to occurred in London, and was under the immediate direction of ſeveral phyſicians of eminence. The uſe of mercury was adopted by my advice; and the eſtimate of the quantity conſumed, as made by the apothecary, has been tranſmitted to me by G. H. Eſq. the father of the child.

is

is carried into the thoracic duct, and there mixed with a large portion of the chyle and lymph, by which its acrimony is ſheathed and diluted, or its chemical properties changed, before it enters the maſs of blood? For the abſorbents of the ſkin, and of the inteſtines, ſhould ſeem to require a capacity to bear the ſtimulus of thoſe extraneous bodies to which, in both ſituations, they are expoſed.

III. MEDICINES INTRODUCED INTO THE COURSE OF CIRCULATION MAY AFFECT THE GENERAL CONSTITUTION OF THE FLUIDS; PRODUCE CHANGES IN THEIR PARTICULAR QUALITIES; SUPERADD NEW ONES; OR COUNTERACT THE MORBIFIC MATTER, WITH WHICH THEY MAY BE OCCASIONALLY CHARGED. By obſervations on the hæmorrhages, which have been ſuſtained without deſtruction to life; from experiments made on animals, by drawing forth all their blood; and by a computation of the bulk of the arteries and veins *(n)*; the maſs of circulating fluids has been eſtimated at fifty pounds, in a middle-ſized man, of which twenty-eight pounds are ſuppoſed to be red blood. Fluids, bearing ſo large a proportion to the weight of the whole body, have aſſuredly very important offices in the animal œconomy. Endued with the common properties of other fluids, they are

(n) Vid. Halleri Prim. Lin. ſect. CXLIX.

ſubject to *mechanical laws*; being variouſly compounded, they are incident to *chemical* changes; and, as they are contained in a living vaſcular ſyſtem, their motions become ſubject to the influence of nervous energy.

But the proſecution of this ſubject will exceed the bounds of the preſent evening's diſcuſſion: And I ſhall reſerve, what I have further to advance upon it, to ſome future meeting of the ſociety.

ESSAY VII.

EXPERIMENTS ON THE SOLVENT POWERS OF CAMPHOR; AND OTHER MISCELLANEOUS COMMUNICATIONS: ADDRESSED TO DR. LETTSOM (*a*).

MANCHESTER, AUGUST 1, 1787.

IF you deem the following facts and observations of sufficient importance to be offered to the Medical Society, I trust they will be received as a small tribute of my respect for an institution, into the fellowship of which I have had the honour of being elected. I do not apologize for the brief and miscellaneous form in which they are delivered, not only because I have no leisure, at this time, for systematic composition, but because I am persuaded this mode of

(*a*) INSERTED in the Memoirs of the Medical Society of London, vol. II. p. 54.

communication is favourable to the advancement of ſcience. It has been adopted by the members of ſeveral foreign academies, and is ſanctioned by the authority of Lord Bacon, and the example of Mr. Boyle. No object or event ſtands ſingle and detached in the great frame of nature. Each has its relations and dependencies, ſimilitudes, contrarieties, and uſes, which a well-informed mind can at once recognize, arrange and purſue; and which increaſing knowledge may multiply to an extent beyond our preſent powers of comprehenſion.

I. I DO not recollect that the SOLVENT POWER OF CAMPHOR, on reſinous ſubſtances, has been particularly noticed by medical writers. It ſeems to be evinced by the following experiments, which I communicate to you, becauſe the reſult of them may be applied to various pharmaceutical uſes.

TEN grains of myrrh were rubbed in a mortar, with two grains of camphor, to which about an ounce of pure water was added, by degrees. The mixture was ſmooth, and the ſediment depoſited, after ſtanding two days, was not conſiderable, and was readily diffuſible again by agitation.

Two grains of camphor were rubbed into a powder, in the mortar; to which an ounce of pure water was gradually added, as in the former experiment. No triture or agitation, as is well known,

known could effect either a solution, or an uniform diffusion.

Two grains of camphor, and the same quantity of myrrh, treated in the like manner, formed a composition sufficiently smooth and equable.

As myrrh is a gummy resinous substance, it is in some degree miscible with water: But in a comparative trial, I found the union much more imperfect than when camphor was combined with it.

These experiments were suggested by the following incident, which lately occurred in my practice. Having directed a composition of camphor and balsam of Tolu, in pills, for a patient going a voyage on account of his health, the apothecary acquainted me that he could not form it into a proper mass; and that it liquified like treacle. The experiment was afterwards made in my presence. At first the two substances would not incorporate, when rubbed together; and I suspected that some *S. V. R.* had been used before, to promote their union. But the triture being continued, a sudden combination and liquefaction took place.

Camphor probably acts as an essential oil, in dissolving resin. When a composition is required of these substances, in a pilular form, it is rendered practicable by the addition of a ſmall portion of the coagulated yolk of an egg.

II. I HAVE preſcribed, with conſiderable ſucceſs, to various patients, a mineral water, which I believe is little known in England. It ſprings from the Hartfell Mountain, about three miles north of Moffatt; and a very full account of it is given by Doctor Horſeburgh, in the firſt volume of the Phyſical and Literary Eſſays. A lady, who had been making a tour in Scotland, brought me a bottle of it, ſome time ago; but I did not examine it, till a caſe of chronic hæmorrhagy, attended by Dr. Eaſon and myſelf, ſuggeſted the trial of ſuch a ſtyptic remedy. The water appears to be a ſtrong chalybeate, and to contain a portion of alum. It is not unpleaſant to the taſte; and, in the doſe of about a quarter of a pint, is grateful to the ſtomach. It relieves uneaſy irritations, and ſlight pains in that organ; promotes digeſtion; and abates flatulence, if taken before meals; and though acidulous in taſte, corrects acidity, and does not even coagulate milk when mixed with it. I have had experience of its efficacy in profuſe diſcharges of the *catamenia*, in the *fluor albus*, in *dyſpepſia*, in *ſtruma*, and other diſorders originating from a laxity of the fibres. In ſuch maladies, chalybeates have been long employed; and Boerhaave, you know, ſpeaks

of

of their virtues with enthuſiaſtic admiration, aſſerting that no medicine, either animal or vegetable; no diet; no regimen can produce the effects, which are accompliſhed by iron. And as I think the Hartfell Spa water is one of the pleaſanteſt forms, under which this active remedy can be adminiſtered, with conſiderable efficacy; as the moſt faſtidious patients may be prevailed upon to take it, when drugs are loathed and neglected; as it is much cheaper, as well as ſtronger, than that of Pyrmont, or Spa; and as it bears carriage without injury, it promiſes to be a valuable acquiſition. Its aluminous impregnation, alſo, adds to the medicinal powers which it poſſeſſes as a tonic, a ſedative, and a ſtyptic. There is often a morbid ſenſibility and irritability in the ſtomach and *primæ viæ*, which render the office of digeſtion uneaſy and painful; and create an habitual diſpoſition to flatulence, and to ſlight attacks of colic. Alum, as I have noticed in a former work, is a valuable remedy under theſe circumſtances. And, combined with iron, by the chemiſtry of nature, its energy, as a ſtyptic, will doubtleſs be increaſed.

III. I LATELY met with an inſtance of *Tuſſis Convulſiva*, ſucceeding the croup, in a boy about three years of age. He was perfectly free from cough, when ſeized with the *Cynanche Trachealis*; and hooped violently when

 that

that diſorder was removed. Are theſe two maladies of the ſame genus? In both there ſubſiſts a ſpaſm of the muſcles of the *glottis*, occaſioning ſymptoms of ſuffocation; and both are moſt effectually relieved by emetics, and antiſpaſmodics, ſuch as the flowers of zinc, James's powder, and muſk.

SUCH a membrane, as is formed in the *trachœa arteria*, is ſometimes generated in the inteſtines. Lady A—— G——, aged two years, had an aphthous fever, during which a few aſcarides appeared in her ſtools. On this account, when ſufficiently recovered, ſhe took a doſe of rhubarb and calomel, which occaſioned the diſcharge of ſix or eight annular ſubſtances, reſembling, in figure, portions of guts, but evidently unorganized. I found them to be nothing more than gluten, ſecreted probably by ſome parts of the alimentary canal, affected by the fever, with aphthous inflammation.

IV. VARIOUS writers, particularly the poets, have ſanctioned the notion, that in the JAUNDICE, objects are painted on the retina of the ſame colour, with that which tinges the external coat of the eye. This I regarded, till lately, as a vulgar error; and endeavoured to ſhew, in a Treatiſe on the Alliance of Natural Hiſtory with Poetry, that it is neither confirmed by experience, nor conſonant to reaſon; and that, in the worſt caſes

cases of the jaundice now known, the symptom has no existence. But two instances have lately occurred, in the circle of my practice, which clearly evince that the opinion has sometimes a foundation in fact; and that conclusions, drawn even from a very general induction, may be fallacious: For my observations were made with attention, during a course of near twenty years. The patients, now alluded to, were men of middle age, who had lived intemperately, whose malady had proved obstinate, but whose eyes were not tinged with bile in an extreme degree. Yet they were uniform in their testimony, that all white objects assumed a yellow cast; and that this hue was deepest on their rising from bed in a morning.

V. A few years ago, a gentleman consulted me about the state of his eyes. He had for a long time felt an uneasy sensation, whenever he viewed any square object; and this malady was then so much increased, that, in playing at whist, he was under the necessity of holding the cards near his eyes, to preclude the sight of their angular points. The pupil of each eye was remarkably contracted, and the *tunica albuginea* slightly inflamed; yet a moderate light was borne without uneasiness. Vision was sufficiently distinct, at all ordinary distances; but I suspected that the field of it was extremely limited; and that the patient, in viewing a quadrangular object, when near, might poſſibly meaſure it by a muſcular exertion of the organ, which gave pain. But of this he did not appear to have any perception; nor could he recollect the date, or account for the origin of his diſorder. He was not a fanciful, or hypochondriachal man; nor did the complaint ſeem to depend on the ſtate of his ſtomach. Some odd aſſociation of ideas, perhaps, at firſt gave riſe to it. The gentleman lives at a diſtance from Mancheſter; and having been only once conſulted by him, I am unacquainted with the termination of this ſingular malady.

ESSAY

ESSAY VIII.

MEDICAL CAUTIONS AND REMARKS;

PARTICULARLY RELATIVE TO

PULMONARY DISORDERS (a).

NE QUID FALSI DICERE AUDEAT; NE QUID VERI NON AUDEAT.

CICERO.

SUCCESS in the alleviation, or removal of pain and ſickneſs, is ſo pleaſing to humanity, that it is always recorded with ſatisfaction, and received with applauſe. We cannot wonder, therefore, at the numerous recitals of it in the annals of phyſic; whilſt diſappointment is rarely mentioned, and error is aſſiduouſly concealed. Yet though the profeſſors of the healing art are acknowledged to hold the firſt rank in erudition, they have aſſuredly no claim to infallibility; nor does it imply diſparagement to aſſert, that the farther their knowledge and experience are enlarged, the

(a) INSERTED in the Memoirs of the Medical Society of London, vol. II. p. 288.

the more they will perceive and lament the imperfection of ſcience, and the inefficacy of medicine. Credulity is often ſucceeded by ſcepticiſm; and the young phyſician, who repeatedly feels his benevolence fruſtrated, and his confidence deceived, may be tempted either to relinquiſh his profeſſion, or ſordidly to purſue it, for the emoluments only which it yields. A candid avowal of ſimilar mortifications, by thoſe who are more advanced in practice, would tend to ſatisfy the mind, to reſtrain unreaſonable expectations of ſucceſs, and even to promote it powerfully, though indirectly, by pointing out the way in which it is not to be attained. Many of the principles of phyſic may be deemed demonſtrative; but the application of them reſts on no other evidence than probability. In different caſes this evidence varies in degree; and we are juſtified in acting according to that degree, which every individual caſe affords. The ſame obſervation may be extended to politics and morality; ſciences which are often clearly underſtood in theory, but egregiouſly miſuſed in the conduct of life. In the ſtudy of the human frame, either corporeal or mental, we proceed analytically, diſſecting the ſeveral parts of which it conſiſts, and diſcriminating their properties, relations, and dependencies. But it is by the contrary proceſs that we form maxims of behaviour,

viour, moral judgments, and therapeutic rules. And it ſometimes requires the moſt comprehenſive knowledge, united with the acuteſt diſcernment, to deduce juſt concluſions from premiſes at once intricate and multifarious. As the philoſopher and politician therefore may, without a bluſh, confeſs their miſtakes concerning characters, actions, and events; ſo the phyſician ought to indulge no apprehenſion of doing injury to his own reputation, or to that of another, by revealing, on proper occaſions, profeſſional diſappointments. Cæſar has related the faults committed by him, in the wars of Gaul. Frederick the Great, of Pruſſia, has followed this noble example of candour and public ſpirit: And Hippocrates, who, as a benefactor to mankind, ranks higher than either of them, records a dangerous error into which he had fallen, that his cotemporaries and poſterity might guard againſt it *(b)*. But without pleading further arguments or authorities, I ſhall lay before the Medical Society a few cautions

(b) À SUTURIS ſe deceptum eſſe Hippocrates memoriæ tradidit, more ſcilicet magnorum virorum, et fiduciam magnarum rerum habentium. Nam levia ingenia, quia nihil habent, nihil ſibi detrahunt. Magno ingenio, multaque nihilominus habituro, convenit etiam ſemper veri erroris confeſſio; præcipueque in eo miniſterio, quod utilitatis cauſa poſteris traditur; ne qui decipiantur eadem ratione, qua quis ante deceptus eſt. Celſ. lib. VIII. cap. 4.

and

and remarks; aſſured of indulgence in that freedom, which is warranted by good intention, and the love of truth.

A PHYSICIAN of probity will feel himſelf accountable for the *omiſſions*, as well as *commiſſions*, which may occur in the courſe of his practice; ſince ſucceſs or dſappointment, recovery or death, may be the reſult of the one, as well as of the other. Several years ago I attended a gentleman, labouring under a peripneumony. He was very corpulent, and the difficulty of breathing and inflammatory ſymptoms required immediate venæſection. The ſurgeon, though a man of ſkill in his profeſſion, twice attempted, without effect, to open a vein in the arm. He then bound up the other arm; but juſt as the point of the lancet was applied to make the orifice, the patient ſtruggled a few ſeconds, and expired. The uſual means of reſtoring animation were tried to no purpoſe; and I was ſhocked with the information, communicated too late, that the gentleman had always a ſtrong dread of phlebotomy; to the terrors of which operation, life, in this inſtance, was probably ſacrificed. So melancholy an example, I truſt, will ever make me attentive to inquire into the feelings and emotions of my patients, in critical circumſtances, as well as into the ſymptoms of their diſeaſes.

WHENEVER

WHENEVER bleeding is thought expedient, in delicate and debilitated ſubjects, which it is too often ſuppoſed to be, in caſes of pulmonary conſumption, if great timidity prevail, it ought to be deemed a ſufficient contraindication. I have ſeen a rigor of ſeveral hours continuance, and extreme proſtration of ſtrength, ſucceed the loſs of only two ounces of blood, in a lady, who dreaded the lancet, though ſhe affected to ſubmit to it with magnanimity. Indeed this very effort might contribute to the injury, by being too great for her feeble frame of mind and body. The like obſervation may be applied to the uſe of voyages in this malady. Such a mean of cure ſhould only be recommended, when there can be full confidence that the patient is equal to the fatigues, and not diſpoſed to be affected by the terrors of it *(c)*. On the ſame grounds of reaſon and humanity, long and painful journeys to

(c) IT has lately been aſſerted, by Doctor Carmichael Smyth in his account of the effects of ſwinging, that the ſea air is prejudicial to the hectic and conſumptive, and even to thoſe who have any tendency to ſuch complaints. In ſome inſtances my experience has been conſonant, in others contradictory to his obſervation. The truth is, *Phthiſis pulmonalis* attacks very different conſtitutions, and originates from different cauſes.

WHEN labouring under a dyſpnœa, many years ago, the conſequence of an hæmoptoe, I went to Scarborough for the benefit of the ſea air. Riding on the beach always irritated

to Briſtol, Matlock, and other places of reſort, are to be adopted with caution. Change of air and of place is often uſeful in this complaint; and I have generally obſerved it to be moſt ſucceſsful, when the *Medicina mentis* has been the principal object of it. There is a languor, an impatience, and irritability, attendant on ſuch invalids, which is wonderfully alleviated by the charms of variety, and the ſoothing influence of rural ſcenery. When a journey therefore is directed, the patient ſhould make frequent ſtops, and reſt ſeveral days at once, in ſuch ſalubrious ſituations, as furniſh comfortable accommodation, and pleaſing views of nature. A plan like this is perfectly compatible with that gentle, moderate regimen of diet and of phyſic, which experience inſtructs us to be moſt appropriate to the ſeveral ſtages of the *phthiſis pulmonalis*. The extreme antiphlogiſtic method of treatment, I have often obſerved to aggravate the ſufferings of the patient, and to accelerate his death. In this malady, inflammation is, perhaps, only an occa-

irritated my lungs, and increaſed the difficulty of breathing. I could ſenſibly perceive the acrimony of the vapours which I inſpired. But on the hills near Scarborough, and on any ſituation where the peculiar odour of the ſhore was not perceptible, I felt refreſhment from every breeze which blew from the ocean.

ſional

ſional concomitant; for the tubercles, in the cellular ſubſtance of the lungs, are found to be of a whitiſh colour and cartilaginous hardneſs, and to remain ſolid till they attain a certain ſize: Matter then begins to be formed in their centre: As they grow larger, ſuppuration advances, till they are converted into *vomicæ*; but theſe retain their white colour and hard texture; and no blood veſſels are to be ſeen upon them, even when examined by a microſcope, after injecting the lungs from the pulmonary artery and vein *(d)*. The ingenious phyſician, to whom we are indebted for ſo intereſting an inveſtigation, hath however informed us, that tubercles, when of a certain bulk, and *vomicæ* alſo, render the portion of the lungs contiguous to them red, ſometimes hard, impervious to air, and conſequently unfit for reſpiration. In the ſtate deſcribed, local inflammation certainly ſubſiſts; yet from long and extenſive experience I have found, that it does not often manifeſt itſelf in the humid climate of Lancaſhire, by ſuch paroxyſms of genuine peripneumonic fever, as require venæſection, or the more active refrigerant medicines. The degree of hectic heat is a fallacious criterion of the propriety of blood-letting; and I have obſerved it to be generally augmented by that eva-

(d) SEE the valuable extracts from Dr. Stark's manuſcript. Medical Communications, vol. I. p. 390.

cuation,

cuation, when the patient is of a ſtrumous habit; when the hair falls off, the nails grow rapidly, and a conſiderable waſting of the fleſh and ſtrength prevails. Under ſuch circumſtances, alſo, I have felt painful diſappointments in the uſe of nitre; the effects of which, as a febrifuge, can only be aſcertained by thoſe, who have had opportunities of attending to its ſubſequent, as well as immediate operation. A youth in my family, ſome time ago, had all the ſymptoms of a true hectic; and as I then entertained a favourable opinion of this remedy, I repeatedly adminiſtered it to him in the doſe of fifteen grains. The pulſe was uſually reduced by it from one hundred and ten, to ninety ſtrokes in a minute, for the ſpace of about a quarter of an hour; that is, whilſt the ſtomach remained ſenſible to the ſedative powers of the ſalt. But a re-action ſoon ſucceeded in the ſyſtem, and the pulſe was frequently quickened to one hundred and thirty vibrations, continuing in the accelerated much longer than in the retarded ſtate; and always ſuffering a permanent diminution of ſtrength. In caſes of this kind, certain medicines of the tonic claſs prove eventually antiphlogiſtic. A young lady, aged ſixteen, nearly related to me, was, in the ſpring of 1785, affected with pulmonic complaints, which threatened a *phthiſis*. As they were accompanied

with

with great languor and debility, I gave her a ſolution of twelve grains of myrrh, every ſix hours, in a ſaline efferveſcing draught, marking the effect on the pulſe with anxious attention. I ſhall tranſcribe from my notes only the firſt obſervation which I made, becauſe each ſubſequent one was ſimilar in reſult. April the 20th, half paſt ſeven o'clock in the evening, pulſe one hundred and twenty, feeble: the draught adminiſtered. Ten minutes before eight, pulſe ninety-eight, ſtronger and fuller; half paſt eight, pulſe one hundred. By perſeverance in the uſe of this remedy, and other auxiliary means, the young lady happily recovered her health and ſtrength. Camphor has been juſtly recommended in the *phthiſis pulmonalis*; but ſhould be given in ſuch ſmall doſes, as not to offend the ſtomach. It combines perfectly with myrrh; and notwithſtanding its ſuppoſed heating quality, perhaps acts rather as a ſedative than ſtimulant on the arterial ſyſtem, as ſeems to be evinced by the following curious fact, communicated to me by my late friend Dr. Dobſon. "In June, 1780, three drachms of camphor were adminiſtered to a maniacal patient, in doſes of one ſcruple, within the ſpace of twenty-four hours. The pulſe was reduced from eighty to ſeventy ſtrokes in a minute, and the *mania* was mitigated. The ſucceeding day, the ſame quantity was given in twelve hours: Profuſe ſweatings and great itching enſued; the pulſe ſunk to fifty-five; and the *mania* was cured." In the treament of pulmonic diſorders, particular attention ſhould always be paid to the reciprocal ſympathy, which ſubſiſts between the ſtomach, the lungs, and the heart. Whatever occaſions an agreeable ſenſation in the organs of digeſtion, and at the ſame time gives a gentle degree of tone to them, will tend to abate the velocity of the pulſe, and to check the violence and frequency of coughing. Porter, on theſe accounts, often proves a grateful and ſalutary beverage; and affords peculiar ſupport and refreſhment under colliquative ſweats *(e)*. But we cannot, from the ſenſible qualities alone of the ſubſtances to be adminiſtered, aſcertain their operation on this delicate organ, liable perhaps, in ſuch affections, to peculiar and anomalous feelings. Indeed the action of moſt medicines on the human body is rather relative than abſolute; and cooling or heating, ſedative or ſtimulant are, in many inſtances, convertible powers, when applied to different maladies, or to diverſified

(e) THE colliquative ſweats, of the *phthiſis pulmonalis*, are much alleviated by the uſe of a calico waiſtcoat or ſhirt, which has been ſteeped in a ſtrong decoction of the bark. It ſhould be well dried, and daily renewed.

ſtates

ſtates of the nervous ſyſtem. A gentleman of rank, in this county, was ſuppoſed to be in an advanced ſtage of what is termed a galloping conſumption, having an inceſſant cough, an expectoration apparently purulent, continued heats, and night ſweats. Yet his cure was accompliſhed, by giving wine whey copiouſly, and by adminiſtering large doſes of ſalt of hartſhorn with ſpermaceti. A very low regimen had been directed by his phyſicians. The cordial one was adopted by degrees, and with a cautious obſervance of its effects; which happily proved to be a progreſſive abatement of the fever, cough, and ſpitting, a gentle fit of the gout, to which the patient had formerly been ſubject, and the perfect re-eſtabliſhment of his health.

In a curious fact, recorded by Dr. Mead, there appears to have been an interchangeable relation between lunacy and the *phthiſis pulmonalis*; the latter being cured by the acceſſion of the former malady, and recurring as ſoon as the brain was reſtored to its natural functions *(f)*. I have

(f) Since this paper was written, the following intereſting fact has occurred in my practice. Mr. C—'s daughter, aged nine years, after labouring under the ſymptoms of *phthiſis pulmonalis* four months, was affected with unuſual pains in her head. Theſe rapidly increaſed to ſuch a degree, as to occaſion frequent ſcreamings. The cough, which had before

 been

I have received authentic information of a ſtate of fatuity, ſubſiſting from infancy, and nearly approaching to ideotiſm, that, after thirty-four years, terminated in a conſumption of the lungs; towards the fatal cloſe of which, the patient diſplayed a degree of intellectual vigour, aſtoniſhing to her family and friends, and not leſs ſo to a learned and judicious clergyman, who viſited her officially, and who communicated this account to me. Indeed, in a true hectic fever, the mental powers are generally in a ſtate of improvement; and it is the lively perception of it, which probably excites thoſe emotions of hope, that afford ſuch ſeaſonable ſupport and conſolation to the ſufferer. Whereas imbecility of mind, when not accompanied with torpor, is always characterized by dejection and deſpair.

The pathology of the pulmonary conſumption is not yet aſcertained, as will appear from a review of the diſcordant opinions of numberleſs writers, from the time of Hippocrates to the preſent period. The following propoſitions may, perhaps,

been extremely violent, and was attended with ſtitches in the breaſt, now abated; and in a few days ceaſed almoſt entirely. The pupils of the eyes became dilated; a *ſtrabiſmus* enſued; and, in about a week, death put a period to her agonies. Whether this affection of the head aroſe from the effuſion of water, or of blood, is uncertain; but its influence on the ſtate of the lungs is worthy of notice.

perhaps, lead to a more ſucceſsful inveſtigation of this intereſting ſubject.

CONSUMPTION, when it originates from what is termed a ſevere cold, is generally preceded by a catarrhal inflammation and fever.

THIS fever ſubſides, but the cough continues; tubercles are formed; and a different ſpecies of fever, or the true hectic, takes place.

THE progreſs to this ſecond ſtage is frequently ſo ſlow and gradual, as not to be much noticed. Yet the hectic ſymptoms, when they occur, are more violent; the proſtration of ſtrength, *maraſmus*, colliquative ſweats, and *diarrhœa*, advance with greater rapidity, and terminate ſooner in death. In ſuch caſes the patients are generally of a ſtrumous habit.

TUBERCLES and *vomicæ*, probably conſtitute the characteriſtics of the diſorder in every form; and in their action they ſeem to bear ſome ſlight analogy to the ulcers, or gangrene of the throat, in the *angina maligna*. They produce a contamination of the parts which are contiguous to them; excite inflammation in the lungs, and a local diſpoſition to *ſphacelus*; generate a purulent matter, often of an acrimonious quality; and deſtroy the vital energy by a fever of a peculiar type.

IN the treatment of *hæmoptyſis*, the antiphlogiſtic plan is now generally adopted in moſt parts of England. And during the incipient ſtage of the diſorder, when the inflammatory diatheſis commonly prevails, much injury may be done by heating ſtyptics and rough aſtringents. But during its progreſs, the type is often changed. And many caſes occur, which, even in their commencement, indicate great laxity of the ſolids and tenuity of the fluids. Under ſuch circumſtances, venæſection, nitre, and the debilitating claſs of medicines, are highly improper, though great authorities have ſanctioned their uſe without ſufficient diſcrimination. When the diſcharge of blood has continued ſome time, a new ſtate of the ſyſtem is induced; the heart and arteries ſeem to loſe their due degree of tone; an increaſed irritability takes place in the ruptured veſſel, and in thoſe which are contiguous to it; and thus the impetus of the circulation is partially augmented, with a diminution of its general energy. Remedies, therefore, which rouſe the vital powers, and excite an equable action in the vaſcular ſyſtem, are clearly indicated. A bliſter, applied to the back, has ſtopped a naſal hæmorrhage. Wine, drunk to intoxication, has cured both *hæmaturia* and *hæmoptyſis*, when other means have failed. And the following fact proves the efficacy of opium, in the malady under conſideration. Mrs. ——, when about thirty-eight years of age, was attacked with an *hæmoptoe.*

hæmoptoe. It was ſuppoſed to originate from violent retchings; and was afterwards increaſed by cloſe confinement, and long attendance on a ſick child. The quantity, diſcharged from the lungs, was from ſix to ten ounces daily, during the ſpace of more than two months. All the uſual means of relief proving ineffectual, and her fleſh and ſtrength declining rapidly, the trial of opium was recommended and happily adopted. She began with taking a grain of thebaic extract every twelfth hour; and by degrees increaſed each doſe to ten grains, ſo that for a long time ſhe had a ſcruple of opium adminiſtered to her daily. The hæmorrhage quickly abated after the commencement of this courſe, and, by perſeverance in it, ceaſed altogether. But on any omiſſion of the uſe of opium, ſhe was threatened with a recurrence of the diſorder; and ſhe has been neceſſitated to continue the remedy for nine years. At this time, Auguſt 1787, ſhe takes ten grains every twenty-four hours.

The uſe of the *pediluvium* in hæmorrhages has often been recommended; but with a reſtriction that its temperature ſhall not exceed ninety-ſix or one hundred degrees of Fahrenheit's thermometer. This prohibition is not well founded, if a ſtimulant be required. When I have occaſion to bathe my feet, for the head-ach, the water, which I uſe, is generally as hot as I can bear it to be;

and the ſenſation which it firſt produces, is that of univerſal chillineſs, attended with *rigor.* A glow of warmth ſucceeds, and afterwards a gentle perſpiration; but the addition of more hot water renews, in a ſlighter degree, a momentary feeling of cold. It is obvious, that ſuch an operation would be favourable in ſome caſes of hæmorrhage. How is the chilling ſenſation to be explained? Does the partial ſtimulus of heat, like that of cold, contract, in its firſt operation, the ſmall cutaneous veſſels?

IN America, the treatment of *hæmoptyſis* widely differs from that which is practiſed in this country. Dr. Ruſh informs me, that common ſalt is the remedy univerſally employed; that it is adminiſtered in large ſpoonfuls, in a dry form; and that its ſalutary effects are ſudden, and for the moſt part certain. In a letter, dated Philadelphia, February 16, 1788, he ſays,

"I AM ſorry to find that you entertain a "ſingle doubt of the ſafety or efficacy of com-"mon ſalt in *hæmoptyſis.* I could ſend you "above a hundred caſes that eſtabliſh both. "My own would be one of them. On the "ſecond of April, 1786, I was ſeized with this "diſorder. It came on in the middle of the "night, and for a while was attended with alarm-"ing ſymptoms. I took a table ſpoonful of "fine Liverpool ſalt, and immediately the

"hæmorrhage

" hæmorrhage was checked. It excited a burn-" ing ſenſation in my throat, that gave me ſome " pain; but this pain was probably part of the " remedy the ſalt afforded. To prevent a re-" turn of the diſorder, as my pulſe was full, I " loſt ten ounces of blood, and lived a few " weeks on a vegetable diet. After this I took " red bark, from which I derived great benefit, " and have never ſince had the leaſt return of " *hæmoptyſis.*"

SALT is frequently applied, in this country, to external wounds as a ſtyptic. In ſpittings of blood, therefore, which originate about the fauces, it may act in the ſame way. But ſuch are not the caſes to which Dr. Ruſh refers; and ſo judicious and experienced a phyſician could not miſtake the ſpurious, for the genuine *hæmoptyſis.* Whether the American practice be adopted amongſt us or not, we ſhall, at leaſt, be warranted by it to urge more circumſpection and diſcrimination, in the uſe of phlebotomy and refrigerants *(g)*.

The

(g) THE action of alimentary ſalt, and of nitre, in large doſes, is very powerful. In a ſingular worm-caſe, recorded by Dr. Heberden (ſee Medical Tranſactions, vol. I. p. 54.) two pounds of common ſalt, diſſolved in two quarts of ſpring water, were taken within the ſpace of an hour. Great oppreſſion of the ſtomach ſoon occurred. Sickneſs, vomiting,

---

The Publication of this Essay, *in the* Memoirs *of the* Medical Society, *occaſioned ſome* Inquiries, *from a very ingenious* Physician, *concerning the Subject of it; to whom the following* Answer *was returned.*

THE young lady, whoſe caſe is briefly deſcribed in the Memoirs of the Medical Society, vol. II. p. 297, (p. 336 of the preceding Eſſay) had no ſtrumous diſpoſition. The uſe of myrrh was continued, many weeks: Geſtation was daily

vomiting, purging, ſweating, rawneſs and ſoreneſs of the alimentary canal, thirſt and ſtrangury enſued. But theſe diſtreſſing ſymptoms were of ſhort continuance. In June 1780, an elderly gentlewoman took about an ounce of nitre, diſſolved in warm water, inſtead of Glauber's ſalts. The *œſophagus, cardia,* and ſtomach, were almoſt inſtantly affected with ſevere pain. In a few minutes ſhe perceived the miſtake which had been made. A ſpoonful of ſweet oil was given; and afterwards repeated draughts of chamomile tea were adminiſtered. Vomiting enſued; and ſhe diſcharged a conſiderable quantity of ſtrongly coagulated, and very ponderous phlegm. The next day I was conſulted, but did not ſee her. The pain in her ſtomach remained. She had a conſtant nauſea, and felt great languor; but had neither *rigor,* ſweating, looſeneſs, nor increaſed diſcharge of urine. Demulcent diet, and a cordial and anodyne mixture ſoon reſtored her health.

employed

employed, when the weather admitted of it: She often drank porter, at her meals: light animal food was allowed: She was ſent into the country, near Mancheſter; and afterwards to a friend's houſe, on the banks of the Merſey, diſtant only a few miles from the ſea. At this time the Peruvian bark was adminiſtered in the form of pills, combined with a little rhubarb and ſalt of tartar, on account of the weakneſs and acidity of her ſtomach.

I HAVE read, with attention and ſatisfaction, your account of a caſe of *phthiſis pulmonalis*, in the London Medical Journal of 1788. But I cannot concur with you in opinion, that debility is to be conſidered, ſolely, as the proximate cauſe of this formidable diſeaſe; though it is ſo univerſally a concomitant, as to render the antiphlogiſtic treatment, in many caſes, unwarrantable, when carried to any extent. Yet I am perſuaded the ſymptoms may be ſuch, as to indicate venæſection. And I have ſeen inſtantaneous relief, obtained from it, when ſevere ſtitches have occurred, and the patient has been in a ſtate of *dyſpnœa*, threatening ſuffocation. The waſte of the fluids not being proportionate to that of the ſolids, and the action of the heart being much diminiſhed, a *plethora* ſeems to be the neceſſary conſequence, which nature often attempts to remedy by ſweats or *diarrhœa*. Bleeding may, therefore,

therefore, be occaſionally expedient, to reſtore the equilibrium between the circulating fluids, and the powers of the vaſcular ſyſtem. But I believe this expediency may, for the moſt part, be confined to particular emergencies; and that the ſame ſalutary end may be more effectually and permanently attained, by ſuch means as augment the vital energy. The tonics, however, which are employed, ſhould be ſuch only, as ſtimulate in the gentleſt degree, otherwiſe the contractions of the heart will become quicker inſtead of ſtronger, the circulation through the lungs will be rendered more imperfect, and the vital powers will ſuſtain a laſting injury.

If it be true that the ſweats, in the *phthiſis pulmonalis*, are efforts of nature, to obviate the proportionate ſuperabundance of the fluids, it will follow that they ſhould not entirely be reſtrained. Indeed they are the criſis of the nocturnal fever, which occurs. And when the patient riſes from his bed ſo early, as to anticipate their coming on, he will experience a ſubſequent aggravation of his moſt diſtreſſing hectic ſymptoms. A *diarrhœa* will alſo be the probable conſequence, which waſtes the ſtrength more than the moſt profuſe ſweatings; not only by carrying off what ſhould be converted into nutriment, but by producing an *atonia* of thoſe organs, whoſe integrity is eſſential to the vigour of the body

body. We ſhould be ſolicitous, therefore, to moderate rather than to ſuppreſs the cutaneous evacuations: A biſcuit ſteeped in wine, a draught of porter, or a doſe of the ſolution of myrrh, now ſo generally uſed, will often ſucceed, when adminiſtered at the commencement of the perſpiration: And after it has continued gently, for ſome time, the patient may change his coverings; riſe from his bed; and he will thus find himſelf rather refreſhed than debilitated by the perſpiration.

A RECOMMENDATION of WINE, in the pulmonary conſumption, will be alarming to many practitioners. But let it be recollected, that it is the moſt efficacious antiphlogiſtic, in the burning fever of the *angina maligna*; and that the ſtomach is familiarized to its ſtimulus, by the daily habit of drinking it at our meals. When it is adminiſtered however to phthiſical patients, the moſt accurate attention ſhould be paid to its effects on the pulſe. Experience will then be our guide, and I believe, if the uſe of it be confined to the period of languor, which always ſucceeds the pneumonic *pyrexia*, we ſhall do good, without incurring the riſque of injury. I have lately had, under my care, a lady, who has been long ſubject to *hæmoptyſis*, and whoſe lungs are ſo delicate, that ſhe ſuffers a relapſe, whenever ſhe breathes a cloſe warm air, for any length

length of time. She has ſtrictly confined herſelf, many years, to a vegetable diet; and finds that even a ſlight indulgence in animal food occaſions a conſiderable degree of fever, and ſometimes a freſh *hæmorrhage.* But ſhe drinks daily, with advantage, ſeveral glaſſes of red port wine. Rheniſh, or old hock, mixed with Seltzer water, forms a pleaſant, cooling, and tonic beverage, in hectical diſorders. Though I have objected to the uſe of nitre, in the paper before referred to, the ſaline mixture, eſpecially when given in the ſtate of efferveſcence, is highly ſalutary, in the febrile paroxyſms of pulmonary conſumption. It produces a grateful ſenſation in the ſtomach, and is ſedative, without being debilitating. Myrrh may very commodiouſly, and with good effects, be combined with it. Indeed I regard this remedy as the moſt uſeful, which modern practice has adopted in conſumptions. Yet when the Rev. Dr. Griffith firſt communicated to me the MS. of his father concerning it, before his Work on Hectic and Slow Fevers was publiſhed, I entertained many doubts of the propriety or even ſafety of adminiſtering it. And before I ventured to follow ſo novel a practice, I conſulted Sir John Pringle; whoſe letter, on the occaſion, I happened to look into, a few days ago. "As for Dr. G's publication, it "was certainly with Sir George Baker's ap-"probation

"probation and mine; though for my part I "had no experience of his medicines, and ſhould "never, from theory, have preſcribed them. "But as the author was believed to be an honeſt "man; and as I have more regard to experi- "ence, and the obſervations of old and plain "phyſicians, than to my own ſpeculations, I "made no difficulty in giving my advice, for "the publication of this little book."—This paragraph I copy, as a pleaſing proof of Sir John Pringle's candour, and as an example worthy of imitation by thoſe, who are wedded, from long habit, to the antiphlogiſtic treatment of the pulmonary conſumption.

In a paper communicated to Dr. Duncan, and inſerted in the Medical and Philoſophical Commentaries, vol. V. p. 166. I have recommended the flowers of zinc, in the diſorder now under our conſideration: And this remedy, though a powerful tonic, neither increaſes heat, nor quickens the vibrations of the pulſe.

Near twenty years ago, in a conſultation which I had with my late excellent friend Dr. Fothergill, on the caſe of a delicate young lady, labouring under the *phthiſis pulmonalis*, I remember he recommended the Buxton waters to her. I objected to the uſe of them, on account of their heating quality, and he was much ſurprized, on being aſſured by me, that they raiſed my my pulſe from eighty to a hundred and nine vibrations in a minute, when taken in a full quantity. But experience has now convinced me, that many medicines, uſually denominated heating, are adminiſtered with advantage, in ſome ſtages of pulmonary conſumption. And as the Buxton water might be ſingularly uſeful in caſes, that originate from intemperance, in which the ſtomach and liver are affected, in conjunction with the lungs, and the patient would ſink into a ſtate of languiſhment and deſpondency, by the ſudden and total diſuſe of what is cordial, I have propoſed the following queries to a judicious practitioner of the place. "Have you ſeen the Buxton water uſed, in the hectical period of *phthiſis pulmonalis?*—What have been its effects?—Have you tried it in the more ſpurious pulmonary conſumption, ariſing from ebriety?—What have been its effects under ſuch circumſtances?"

THE anſwer, which I have received, is, in ſubſtance, as follows. "In all the caſes, which "have fallen under my obſervation of genuine "*phthiſis*, and in all the ſtages of that diſorder, "the Buxton waters have appeared to me to "be injurious. On the contrary I have ſeen the "beſt effects produced by them, in various "caſes, where the ſtomach has been impaired by "ebriety; where the liver has been affected; "and

" and a bad cough has attended, together with " a copious and even purulent expectoration. " Such cafes I have, again and again, feen won- " derfully relieved by the ufe of our waters."

In treating on a fubject fo interefting to the profeffion, and which has often engaged my ferious and very anxious attention, I have gone into a much longer detail, than was my defign, when I fat down to write to you. I fhall therefore haften to relieve you and myfelf, from the prolixity of this letter, by offering my beft wifhes for the fuccefs of your undertaking, and by expreffing my hope that a due medium may be happily pointed out, between the *extremes of the cooling and of the heating regimen.*

MANCHESTER, MAY 25, 1789.

ESSAY IX.

OBSERVATIONS

ON THE MEDICINAL USES OF THE

OLEUM JECORIS ASELLI,

OR COD LIVER OIL,

IN THE

CHRONIC RHEUMATISM, AND OTHER PAINFUL DISORDERS (a).

THE multiplicity of articles, which constitutes the *Materia Medica*, has been a subject of complaint with some physicians: And though it is an evil of no great magnitude, it certainly requires correction and reformation. For it must be acknowledged that many of them are known only by their names; and that others are so seldom prescribed, as scarcely to merit the places, which they retain in the officinal lists. The progressive accumulation, however, of inactive remedies, is not to be deemed

(a) Inserted in the London Medical Journal, vol. III. p. 393.

introduction

an argument againſt, but an incitement to the introduction of new ones, which are more efficacious. And, I truſt, it will be doing ſome ſervice to the healing art, to communicate to the public a brief account of the *Oleum jecoris aſelli*, or cod liver oil; the ſalutary properties of which, I believe, have been little experienced beyond the vicinage of Mancheſter.

THIS medicine is diſpenſed ſo largely in the hoſpital here, that near a hogſhead of it is annually conſumed. It is given in obſtinate chronic rheumatiſms, ſciaticas of long ſtanding, and in thoſe caſes of premature decrepitude, which originate from immoderate labour, repeated ſtrains and bruiſes, or expoſure to continual dampneſs and cold; by which the muſcles and tendons become too rigid, and the flexibility of the joints is impaired, ſo as to crackle for want of a due ſecretion of *ſynovia*. While I was one of the phyſicians to this charity, I had the fulleſt evidence of the ſucceſsful exhibition of cod liver oil, in various maladies, of the claſs above deſcribed, which had reſiſted other powerful modes of treatment. And I frequently compared its operation with that of gum guaiacum, by preſcribing each, at the ſame time, to different patients in ſimilar circumſtances. Theſe trials almoſt always terminated in favour of the oil; and the patients, who took guaiacum, by conferring with their fellow-ſufferers, were ſometimes ſo ſenſible of making a ſlower progreſs towards recovery, as to requeſt a change of one remedy for the other.

At firſt it occaſions, for the moſt part, an increaſe of pain; but this effect ſhortly ceaſes, and a gradual abatement of the ſymptoms ſucceeds. The pulſe, in irritable habits, is ſometimes accelerated by it, and a glow of warmth has been felt through the whole body, after each doſe of the medicine. It is neither uniformly laxative, nor binding; but often promotes a gentle degree of perſpiration. However, it proves ſucceſsful, even when it produces no ſenſible operation, as generally happens in perſons habituated to its uſe. In a few weeks, the appetite is impaired by it, the tongue grows foul, and an emetic is required. The doſe of it varies from one table-ſpoonful to three, and it may be adminiſtered twice, thrice, or four times daily. In many caſes, it is found ſerviceable to rub the parts affected, with the oil, during the courſe of its internal exhibition. But this practice is only to be followed, when no great ſoreneſs ſubſiſts. Indeed, either fever or inflammation forbids the uſe of it entirely.

Cod liver oil is chiefly brought from Newfoundland. It forms a conſiderable article of merchandize; and comes in barrels from 400 to 520lb.

520lb. in weight. The method of obtaining it is, by heaping together the livers of the fiſh, from which, by a gentle putrefaction, the oil flows very plentifully. A ſimilar oil is procured from the livers of the fiſh called ling, and alſo from a ſmall ſpecies of cod, found on the coaſt of Buchan in the north of Scotland. The taſte is nauſeous, and leaves upon the palate a ſavour, like that of tainted fiſh. On this account, it is not much preſcribed here, in private practice, amongſt the higher orders of people: But the hoſpital patients make no complaints of it; and ſuch is their confidence in its efficacy, that they often ſolicit, as I before obſerved, to take it; and generally perſevere, with ſteadineſs, in the uſe of it. Indeed we know, that oil, of the ſame kind, forms no inconſiderable part of the food of the Laplanders, and other northern nations. For habit ſoon reconciles to the taſte the moſt diſguſting viands. The cod liver oil may, however, be rendered much leſs offenſive by the following mode of adminiſtering it. R. *Ol. Jecoris Aſelli unciam unam, Aq. Menth. Pip. Simp. ſemunciam, Lixiv. Sapon. gutt. XL. Miſce; fiat Hauſtus.* By this combination a liquid ſoap, not very unpleaſant, is produced, which may be readily decompoſed by the addition of a tea-ſpoonful of the juice of lemons. And as the oil is probably moſt efficacious in its original form, it may be

 adviſable

advifable to drink a cup of fome acidulous liquor, immediately after the medicine has been fwallowed. This will at once cleanfe the mouth and gullet, neutralize the alkaline falt, and feparate the oil in the ftomach. Dr. Ruffel, in his Natural Hiftory of Aleppo, has obferved, that "in "certain feafons, when oil is plentifully taken, "the people there become difpofed to fevers "and infarctions of the lungs, which fymptoms "wear off by retrenching this indulgence." I have never feen or heard of any fuch effects, from the long continued ufe of the *oleum jecoris afelli*. Perhaps this diverfity may partly depend on the different qualities of vegetable and fifh oil; the former having a tendency to obftruct, the latter to promote infenfible perfpiration. But, I apprehend, it is chiefly to be afcribed to the influence of climate. The intenfe heats of Turkey relax the animal fibres, and oil adds to this relaxation. But, under a northern fky, the fibres are too much difpofed to rigidity; and when this actually fubfifts, as a malady, the emollient powers of oil are fo far from being injurious, that they are highly falutary.

As my chief defign, in announcing the virtues of the *oleum afelli*, is to recommend its ufe in hofpitals, difpenfaries, and parifh work-houfes, I fhall fubjoin the following letter, written, at my defire, by Mr. Darbey, houfe-furgeon and apothecary

apothecary to our infirmary. The teſtimony which it bears in favour of this medicine, is the more forcible, as it is founded not on the experience of one, but of all the phyſicians to the charity; whoſe patients he daily attends and examines. And it is but juſtice to him to add, that he is a man of judgment, obſervation, and integrity.

"To Dr. PERCIVAL.

"DEAR SIR,

"In compliance with your requeſt, I ſend "you the following remarks on ſome rheumatic "caſes:

"For ſeveral years after I came to the in-"firmary, I obſerved that many poor patients, "who were received into the infirmary for the "chronic rheumatiſm, after ſeveral weeks trial "of a variety of remedies, were diſcharged with "little or no relief. The volatile tincture of "guaiacum, in large doſes, ſeemed to bid the "faireſt to effect a cure; but the ſucceſs did "not anſwer expectation. About ten years "ſince, an accidental circumſtance diſcovered "to us a remedy, which has been uſed with "the greateſt ſucceſs, for the above complaint, "but is very little known, in any county, except "Lancaſhire: It is the cod, or ling liver oil.

 "A WOMAN,

"A WOMAN, who laboured under the moſt "excruciating rheumatiſm, and was an out-"patient of this infirmary, being adviſed to rub "her joints with the oil, was induced to take it, "at the ſame time, internally. A few weeks "reſtored her to the uſe of her limbs, and ſhe "was cured. However, little attention was "paid to this caſe, as it was ſuppoſed that the "alteration of the weather, and the medicines "ſhe had before taken, had cauſed the cure. "About a twelvemonth afterwards, her com-"plaints returned with double violence, and the "ſame remedy reſtored her to health again.

"ENCOURAGED by this ſecond recovery, Dr. "Kay, one of the phyſicians to the infirmary, "preſcribed it for other patients, in ſimilar caſes; "and it anſwered his moſt ſanguine expectations. "Since then it has been uſed by the other "phyſicians, with the greateſt ſucceſs. One "diſadvantage attending the uſe of the fiſh oil "is, its nauſeous ſmell and taſte: This is ſo bad, "that, I am afraid, many delicate ſtomachs "cannot take it. Yet I have obſerved that the "poor, after taking a few doſes, readily drink "it without any appearance of nauſea; and that "not more than one ſtomach in twenty rejects it. "This medicine has very different effects on "different conſtitutions: On ſome it operates "as a purgative; others are coſtive with it; and "ſometimes

" ſometimes it occaſions a gentle ſweat. When " the latter has been the caſe, the cure has been " more certain and expeditious; though it muſt " be obſerved, that the uſe of it, for the firſt " week or fortnight, ſeems to occaſion a general " increaſe of pain.

" MEN and women, advanced in years, whoſe " fibres may be ſuppoſed to have acquired a " degree of rigidity, find ſurprizing effects from " it. Some, who have been cripples for many " years, and not able to move from their ſeats, " have, after a few weeks uſe of it, been able " to go with the aſſiſtance of a ſtick; and, by a " longer continuance, have enjoyed the pleaſing " ſatisfaction of being reſtored to the natural " uſe of their limbs, which, for a long time " before, had been a burden to them.

" Two caſes occurred lately, in which the oil " had an extraordinary effect, even on young " perſons, whoſe ages did not exceed ten years. " Guaiacum, calomel, bliſters, &c. were tried " on both theſe patients, but with ſo little benefit, " that opiates were given, merely to procure tem- " porary eaſe. Their lower limbs ſeemed to be " a burden to them, and they had ſuch an ap- " pearance of diſtortion, that no hopes of relief " could be well entertained. In compliance " with the particular requeſt of their parents, " the cod oil was given: The one obtained a " perfect

" perfect cure, the other nearly so; the latter, " having a little distortion in his back, is pre-" vented the free use of his legs. So general " has been the use of the oil with us, that we " dispense fifty or sixty gallons annually; and " the good effects of it are so well known " amongst the poorer sort, that it is particularly " requested by them for almost every lameness. " Except bark, opium, and mercury, I believe " no one medicine in the *Materia Medica* is likely " to be of greater service. Besides, there is one " other circumstance which recommends this " medicine, which is, that it is a cheap one: " And I could wish for a more general use of it, " in order to prove that the above account of " its good effects is no exaggeration.

" I am, SIR,

" Your obliged humble servant,

" ROBERT DARBEY."

MANCHESTER INFIRMARY,
FEB. 12, 1782.

ESSAY

ESSAY X.

HINTS TOWARDS THE INVESTIGATION OF THE NATURE, CAUSE, AND CURE OF THE RABIES CANINA:

Addreſſed to Dr. HAYGARTH.

MANCHESTER, MAY 1, 1789.

YOUR propoſal, my dear friend, for obviating the baneful effects of the bite of a mad dog, communicated Nov. 17, 1788, claimed my immediate attention; and I wrote to you by the ſubſequent poſt, that no delay might take place in the execution of your benevolent project *(a)*. I have ſince read and thought

(a) COPY *of Dr.* HAYGARTH'S PROPOSAL *for obviating the Effects of the* BITE *of a* MAD DOG.

NEAR Wrexham, in North Wales, three men died of canine madneſs in October and November, 1788.

THESE melancholy caſes ſpread a general alarm. But it ought to give great comfort and ſatisfaction to any one who may

thought much on the ſubject; and ſhall now tranſmit to you the reſult of my better information, and more deliberate reflection. To your candour

may be bitten, to know that there is a ſafe, eaſy, and effectual method of preventing infection; which can ſeldom give pain, or require ſkill, and is in the power of every perſon to employ. It is univerſally allowed by phyſicians, that the ſpittle of a mad animal, infuſed into a wound, is the *only* cauſe hitherto known, that can communicate canine madneſs to the human body. This poiſon does no immediate miſchief, but is ſlowly abſorbed into the blood; and ſufficient opportunity is given to remove it, before any danger can ariſe. Whenever any perſon is bitten, the plain and obvious means of preventing any future injury, is, firſt, to wipe off the ſpittle with a dry cloth, and then to waſh the wound with cold water; not ſlightly and ſuperficially, but abundantly, and with the moſt perſevering attention; in bad caſes, for ſeveral hours. After a plentiful affuſion of cold water, but not ſooner, warm water may be employed with ſafety and advantage: A continued ſtream of it, poured from the ſpout of a tea-pot or tea-kettle, held up at a conſiderable diſtance, is peculiarly well adapted to the purpoſe. If the canine poiſon infuſed into a wound were of a peculiar colour, as black, like ink, we ſhould all be aware that plenty of water and patient diligence would effectually waſh out the dark die; but this could not be expected by a ſlight and ſuperficial ablution. After a bite has been carefully waſhed, colour it with ſaliva, tinged by ink, &c. When ſome hours have elapſed waſh out the ſtain. A viſible proof may thus be obtained, how ſoon and perfectly water can cleanſe a wound from ſaliva. As a proof that ſlight waſhing of the wound is not ſufficient to cleanſe it effectually from the poiſon, we may

candour I can lay myſelf open without reſerve; and from your judgment I ſhall be equally

may mention, that, in ſome caſes, after inoculation for the ſmall-pox, the poiſonous matter has been attempted to be waſhed out of the wound, by perſons who wiſhed to prevent its effects: yet the inoculated ſmall-pox appeared at its proper period. Theſe unſucceſsful attempts were performed ſecretly, haſtily, and timidly, by a female hand. But in a caſe where the inoculated inciſions were probably waſhed with greater care, infection was prevented. Such facts teach us the importance of patient perſeverance in waſhing away the poiſon; but they need not abate our confidence that ſuch perſeverance will certainly be ſucceſsful.

THE ablution ſhould be accompliſhed with great diligence and without delay; and may be performed by the patient or any aſſiſtant. However, as the apprehenſion of this dreadful diſorder always excites the greateſt anxiety, a ſurgeon's advice and aſſiſtance ought to be obtained, as ſoon as poſſible, in all caſes where the ſkin is injured. He will execute theſe directions moſt dexterouſly and completely. In a bad wound, the poiſon may be conveyed deep into the fleſh, by long teeth or lacerations. In ſuch circumſtances he ſhould open and waſh every ſuſpicious place. And, whenever any painful uncertainty can remain, he ſhould cup and ſyringe. If the bite have been neglected, till the inflammation begins, he ſhould, after ſhaving off the inflamed ſurface, cup, ſyringe, and waſh with double diligence. By this method of purification, it cannot be doubted that every particle of poiſon, and, conſequently, that every cauſe of danger may be effectually removed.

[N. B. Let this paper be *paſted* up in ſome public places, and in the houſes of ſeveral ſenſible and humane perſons in each pariſh.]

happy

happy to receive either the correction or confirmation of the following suggestions, relative, I. TO THE NATURE AND CAUSE; II. TO THE PREVENTION; AND III. TO THE CURE OF HYDROPHOBIA.

I. I DO not perceive any strict analogy between the action of the canine virus and that of the *lues venerea*, of the small-pox, or of the viper. These evidently affect the lymphatic system; and their progress into the course of circulation may be readily traced, which is not the case with the poison of a mad dog. Are we then fundamentally right in the idea, that the bite of a rabid animal operates by absorption? Might not its effects be, at least as well if not better, explained by ascribing them to local nervous irritation; propagated, in different periods of time, according to the varying circumstances of sensibility and irritability, to the brain, and from thence to the *fauces*, gullet, and stomach? Are not all the symptoms induced of the nervous and spasmodic class? Or, do any marks appear, in the human kind, of a specific vitiation of the fluids?

THERE seems to be a striking resemblance, in many particulars, between some species of *tetanus* and the *rabies canina (b)*. Now, *tetanus* is known

(*b*) DR. CURRIE, of Liverpool, informs me, that in a case of this disease (*tetanus*) in which wine proved an effectual known to be produced, in certain ſtates of the body, by local irritation, without the leaſt ſuſpicion of any abſorption of poiſon, or contamination of the fluids.

tual remedy, it could only be ſwallowed at certain moments of diminiſhed conſtriction. At other times, if it was ſhewn to the ſufferer, the ſight produced evident diſtreſs; and if it was advanced towards his mouth, it never failed to bring on convulſion. The proper ſeaſon for adminiſtering it was learnt from the patient's ſignal, as he ſpoke with great difficulty: And with every precaution, deglutition was interrupted twice out of three times, that it was attempted, by the acceſſion of convulſion. The wound, which gave riſe to the diſeaſe, was ſo ſlight and ſo nearly healed, that it had eſcaped the patient's notice. If it had eſcaped the notice of the attendants alſo, and if they had been unacquainted with the actual appearance of *tetanus*, my very judicious friend conceives it poſſible, that the diſeaſe might have been named *Hydrophobia*.

The following narrative, which is of a ſimilar kind, I received from Dr. Darwin. A young man had his ankle much torn and bruiſed by a fall from two horſes, which he rode at the ſame time, ſtanding upright, on their backs. In a few days, a difficulty of deglutition occurred, and he became totally convulſed, on attempting to ſwallow fluids. Two open ulcers, near the ankle, were then laid into one: The operation however was in vain. Amputation was then propoſed, but rejected: And in ſpite of the uſe of much opium, and mercurial friction, about the fauces, he died on the ſucceeding day. In this caſe, the doctor juſtly obſerves, the *hydrophobia* was evidently produced by ſympathy with the wounded parts.

MENTAL

Mental impreſſions have repeatedly excited hydrophobia. Some time ago, I attended a clergyman, who laboured under many of the ſymptoms of it, through the ſhock occaſioned by an official viſit, to one of his pariſhioners, dying of that diſeaſe. He had no opinion of the Ormſkirk powder, but the Tonquin remedy (muſk, cinnabar, &c.) perfectly cured him. As Phyſician Extraordinary to our Infirmary, my advice is ſometimes called for on particular occaſions. I was not long ſince conſulted about a man, bitten by a ſuppoſed mad dog. He had the uſual affections of the diſeaſe, though in a ſlight degree, which were removed by mercurials and antiſpaſmodics. When the man was recovered, and qualified to ſtate minutely, and without anxiety, the circumſtances antecedent to his attack; I was perfectly convinced that his malady had originated ſolely from the terrors of imagination. In ſuch caſes, there can, aſſuredly be no ground to impute the malady to the abſorption of any poiſon; and it muſt be aſcribed entirely to nervous irritation.

The accurate Morgagni has related a caſe of hydrophobia, occaſioned by the bite of an enraged cat, which was not mad. The *virus* in this caſe, if *virus* is to be ſuppoſed, could not be of the ſpecific kind belonging to an hydrophobic animal. And the ſymptoms are to be accounted

for

for in the ſame way, in which we explain the conſequences of a wounded tendon, or the ſplinter of a fractured bone, when ſuch cauſes produce a locked jaw or *tetanus*.

The *virus* of the ſmall-pox, or of the *lues venerea* very rarely fails of producing its baneful effects on the body, when applied. Whereas the bite of a mad animal is not found to be deleterious in a very large, though indeterminate number of caſes. Is not ſuch a difference thus explicable? The former is tranſmitted into the ſyſtem by abſorption, through a ſeries of veſſels, which are uniform and regular in their action. The latter is, perhaps, poiſonous only to certain nerves, under certain conditions; ſo that the chance is always great againſt its operation. Juſt ſo it is with wounds or injuries of the tendons: Theſe are very rarely ſucceeded by a locked jaw, and only under peculiar circumſtances.

That a nerve is capable of irritation, independently of the brain, whilſt the vital energy ſubſiſts, is evinced by the contractions of the heart, produced by pricking or wounding it, when taken out of the body. May not this be the power, which is firſt excited by the canine poiſon; and which requires an indefinite time to operate, before it communicates with the brain, or rouſes the perception of injury done to the ſyſtem?

 We

We are informed by a celebrated anatomiſt (Monro), that the nerves reſemble the brain in ſtructure; and that, as they proceed in their courſe, they acquire additional energy.

MORGAGNI aſſerts, that the poiſon of a mad animal has been known to remain latent even for twenty years, till being excited into action by ſome cauſe, certain deſtruction was the conſequence. This information, however, he delivers, not on his own authority, but as what he believes to be founded in truth. Whatever doubt may be entertained of its credibility, there can be none of the caſe, which the ſame author relates, of a boy under his own inſpection, in whom the ſymptoms of the *hydrophobia* came on five months after a bite in the leg, by an animal not then known to be mad. And Dr. Vaughan has given us lately the hiſtory of a patient, who was bitten in September, without any appearance of canine infection till the ſixth of June following. It is evident, therefore, that the injury done may long remain topical, and ſo ſlight as not to be perceived. This occurs in affections confeſſedly originating in the nerves *(c)*.

A DIFFICULTY

(c) SOME time ſince, I attended a lady, who had received a bruiſe on the *os ſacrum*, by a fall, when ſhe was young. She ſoon recovered from its effects: But eighteen years afterwards, the rheumatiſm fixed on the part, was attended

A DIFFICULTY in ſwallowing liquids, or the dread of water is not always a concomitant of the other ſymptoms, incident to perſons bitten by mad animals. This only ſhews a variation in different ſubjects, in the ſympathetic powers of the nervous ſyſtem. And I have lately met with an equal degree of diverſity in an affection of the jaw, produced by an injury from a bodkin in the tendons of the hand. The wound ſoon healed without any inflammation remaining; the pain was not conſtant, nor at any time intenſe. No ſtiffneſs was felt in the jaw; but, on the contrary, a weakneſs and inability to prevent its dropping. The lady chewed and ſwallowed with eaſe; but on reading aloud, ſhe had a pain in the maxillary articulation: Nor could ſhe prevent frequent yawning. This patient had been long an invalid, previous to the accident; and there was reaſon to ſuſpect, in her caſe, ſome antecedent morbid affection both of the brain and of the ſpinal marrow.

DISSECTIONS have hitherto thrown little or no light on the nature of the *rabies canina.* Morgagni, though he has related many hiſtories,

attended with unuſually excruciating pain, and long reſiſted the remedies, commonly employed with much more ſpeedy ſucceſs in that diſorder. In this caſe, we may preſume, there ſubſiſted a morbid topical affection of the nerves, which a ſubſequent cauſe rendered manifeſt.

 declines

declines to draw any conclufion from them; obferving from a comparifon of all, that the dead differ much more from each other than the living. We muft therefore be content with conjecture; and adopt with diffidence that hypothefis, which appears moft confonant to reafon and to truth. And this muft be our clue in the treatment of perfons who may be, or who are actually fufferers by the bite of rabid animals: For we have yet to learn that mode of practice, on the fuccefs of which we can place any juft dependence. Your propofal, therefore, of a more likely mean of *prevention* than any yet fuggefted, merits the cordial thanks of the public.

II. Agreeably to the rules of your printed paper, let the patient, with as much expedition as poffible, wipe off the fpittle of the dog with a dry cloth, (fuppofe his handkerchief, as being always at hand) and then, abundantly and with the moft perfevering attention, wafh the wound with water. The preference you give to *cold* water, for the firft ablution, is judicious; and accords with the idea, above advanced, that the nerves are the parts alone injured by the canine *virus*. They may thus perhaps be rendered torpid, and the *virus* may be greatly diluted or wafhed away, before they recover fuch fenfibility as to be capable of fuffering from its action. Ligatures, placed above and below the

wound

wound, would contribute to the benumbing action of the cold water *(d)*. When this has been sufficiently applied, *warm* water should be used, not only as a better solvent, but to produce a flow of blood; which, coming from numberless small vessels, may tend to complete the cleansing of the wound *(e)*. At this time the cupping-glass would be a good auxiliary *(f)*.

WHEN the part bitten may be supposed to be as much freed from the poison as can be accomplished by ablution, additional security may, perhaps, be afforded by bathing it very well with the gastric juice of a healthy animal, recently killed. The penetrating quality of this fluid; its energy as an almost universal solvent; and its power of rendering even poisons not only innocent, but nutritious, promise a salutary operation under the circumstances described. If we are to expect an antidote to the canine *virus*, this fluid seems more likely to prove such, than any other substance yet discovered. For I have some where

(d) FROM the experiments of Abbé Fontana, concerning the bite of the viper, it appears, that ligatures, round the bitten limb, had a very salutary effect.

(e) PLUNGING the part, infected with the poison of a viper, into *warm* water, and keeping it therein some time, appeared to Abbé Fontana to be truly advantageous.

(f) *Vid.* Cels. lib. VII. cap. 23. § 3.

 seen

ſeen it recorded as a fact, that a piece of meat, imbued with the ſaliva of a mad dog, has been ſwallowed by another dog with impunity. The gaſtric juice of a carnivorous is more active than that of a graminivorous animal. A cat, a dog, or carrion crow may therefore be killed for the purpoſe. From the laſt, Abbé Spallanzani obtained this fluid in great purity, without injury to the bird, by introducing bits of dry ſponge into the ſtomach.

If the gaſtric juice be not attainable, probably the ſaliva of a healthy young perſon would be the beſt ſubſtitute; and it might be procured by the chewing of rennet, which has been well freed from the ſalt *(g)*. We are informed by Celſus, that the Pſylli ſucked, without injury, the poiſon infuſed by ſerpents. The ſpittle is demulcent, inviſcating, and capable of changing the qualities of bodies by its fermentative nature. One or other of theſe applications muſt therefore be renewed

(g) The rennet cannot be entirely freed from the ſalt, with which it is preſerved, without depriving it of a conſiderable portion of gaſtric juice. Perhaps the ſalt itſelf may have ſome ſalutary powers. Abbé Raynal aſſerts, that it counteracts the poiſon of the American Manchineel tree, vol. V. p. 369. Celſus recommends it in the bite of a viper, lib. V. 27. In Virginia, when the Indians are bitten by a rattle ſnake, they lay to the part affected the *radix Senekæ*, well chewed, by which it muſt be fully impregnated with ſaliva. See Mead's Works, p. 44.

ſeveral

ſeveral times daily; and the part ſhould be afterwards covered with a cataplaſm.

In recommending the ſeveral foregoing means of prevention, I would not be underſtood to preclude exciſion of the part bitten, when the patient has courage to undergo the operation, and it can be accompliſhed without danger. But much time may be loſt, before the ſurgeon arrives; the ſufferer may long reſiſt all ſolicitations to ſubmit to the knife; the wound may have been inflicted on the face, or near ſome large blood veſſel; or there may be ſo little probability of the madneſs of the dog, as to render it unjuſtifiable to ſubject the patient to preſent pain, and future deformity. In all theſe caſes, your plan of ablution promiſes much benefit; is liable to no objections; may be inſtantly executed; and will allow ſufficient leiſure for a careful and complete exciſion. The application of cauſtics has been found unſucceſsful: And the exploſion of gun-powder could hardly take place in a bleeding wound: Nor could we ſecure its extenſion through the oblique courſe of the animal's teeth. To this laſt conſideration you have judiciouſly paid attention, by directing water to be poured on the wound from the ſpout of a tea-kettle.

On the ſuppoſition, that the *hydrophobia* is a diſeaſe of the nervous claſs, the means to obviate its accefs fhould feem to be fuch as diminifh fenfibility and irritability, and give tone and vigour to the fyftem. Bark, fteel, *cuprum ammoniacum*, or flowers of zinc may therefore be adminiftered; and the patient fhould be directed to ufe the cold bath frequently. If his mind be agitated, or depreffed, laudanum will occafionally be required. I have reafon to think, that the late Mr. Hill, of Ormfkirk, in fome cafes, joined opiates with his once celebrated fpecific. To the ufe of this popular noftrum, if the patient entertain much confidence in it, there can be no reafonable objection; becaufe only a few dofes of it are recommended, and confequently it cannot long interfere with the exhibition of other more active medicines. Perhaps it may be degraded in the eftimation of the faculty, by not being adminiftered in adequate quantities, or with fufficient perfeverance. To infallibility no remedy yet known can have any juft pretenfions: And the inftances of the failure of the Ormfkirk powder are not more numerous, than thofe which have been recorded of every other mean hitherto employed. It is indeed compofed of ingredients of no great efficacy, in ordinary cafes, fo far as we can rely on the analyfis which has been given of it. But activity or inertnefs are relative, not abfolute qualities, in medicinal fubftances; and their energies, with refpect respect to the human body, depend on the state of the animal system, at the period when they are administered. Experience, therefore, is the only test of their inefficiency or power. In other cases, we find that apparently simple means produce very salutary effects. Thus milk is an useful solvent, when arsenic has been received into the stomach. And I have been informed, by a gentleman of knowledge and veracity, that, in South Carolina, he has seen the poison of the rattle snake speedily counteracted by the juice of plantane and horehound *(h)*. I have enlarged

(h) THIS gentleman was on a visit, in South Carolina, when a servant was bitten in the hand by a rattle snake. Ligatures were instantly applied near the part, but the hand and arm swelled; the jaw became somewhat locked; and the man appeared to be in a state of considerable danger. The surgeon administered to him, by spoonfuls, at short intervals, the juice of plantane and horehound; and the wounded part was covered with a cataplasm of the same herbs bruised. The salutary effects of these remedies were soon apparent; and the servant afterwards perfectly recovered. Mr. Catesby is of opinion, that no remedy is yet discovered for the bite of a rattle snake. Yet he acknowledges the having seen recoveries, but imputes them to the efforts of nature and to the slightness of the bite. How far this may be true of the case above related I shall not attempt to decide; but the observation reminds me of an important distinction, made by Boerhaave, on the comparative danger of infection by a mad dog, under the different stages of his malady.

SINCE

larged on this topic, not from any degree of faith in the powers of the Ormſkirk powder, as an antidote to the canine poiſon; but to obviate pre-

SINCE this paper was written Dr. Darwin has obligingly communicated to me a paſſage, from Abbé Groſier's Deſcription of China, (vol. I. p. 279.) in which it is ſaid, "That people "are often bitten by ſerpents, at Tang-king, and are cured "by applying to the wound, a ſtone reſembling a cheſnut, "which is called ſerpent ſtone. The ſtone, after preſſing "out the blood, is applied to the wound, to which it ad- "heres, ſucking out the poiſon, and then falls off. It is "then well waſhed in lime water and dried, and applied a "ſecond time to the wound: Or another ſtone may be uſed. "And thus the poiſon is extracted." Whether the Abbé's obſervations may be relied upon, it is not eaſy to decide; but certain it is, that an abſorbent earth acts forcibly, by the attraction of capillary tubes; as any one may experience by holding a freſh burnt tobacco pipe between the lips. The poiſoned wound, however, muſt be both recent and ſuperficial, to be cleanſed by ſuch a remedy. The Bramins of India expoſe to ſale an antidote, which they pretend to be taken out of the head of the hooded ſerpent. Redi, however, aſſerts that it is made of calcined hartſhorn, which is an active abſorbent. On this occaſion you will recollect the fact lately tranſmitted to you by Dr. Waterhouſe, profeſſor of phyſic at Cambridge, in New England, that when a rattle ſnake bites the noſe of a dog, he digs a hole in the ground, lays his head in it, and is commonly cured. It is probable that the ſurface of the earth is in a very aduſt and conſequently abſorbing ſtate, in thoſe parts of America, where ſuch accidents occur; and that the noſe of this animal is leſs ſuſceptible of being injured by poiſon, from its coldneſs, and from the ſlime with which it is covered, than any other part of the body.

poſſeſſions

poſſeſſions, which miſlead inveſtigation, and obſtruct the attainment of a ſuccesſful remedy, in this moſt dreadful of human diſorders.

III. THE acceſſion of canine madneſs is uncertain as to the diſtance of time from the bite; and the ſymptoms by which it firſt manifeſts itſelf. But frequently the *cicatrix* becomes hard and elevated; pains ſhoot from it towards the head; it is ſurrounded with livid or red ſtreaks; and the wound breaks out afreſh. The friends of the patient ſhould be apprized of the appearances which are to be ſuſpected, that they may be ſedulouſly watchful, and give inſtant notice, to the medical practitioner employed, of the change which has occurred. In this firſt ſtage of the diſeaſe, a large doſe of thebaic extract ſhould be adminiſtered, to obtain, if poſſible, a truce. This remedy ſeems appropriate to various ſymptoms of the *hydrophobia*; and we might have hoped it would have merited our entire reliance, from Mr. Pott's aſſurances of its great efficacy, in the painful mortification of the toes, which is ſomewhat analogous, in its commencement. But experience has ſhewn that it produces no laſting benefit. And recourſe muſt be had, without delay, to ſome other medicine, adequate to counteract the impreſſion of the canine poiſon, by another impreſſion, equally forcible,

forcible, on the nervous ſyſtem *(i)*. The qualities of the FOX-GLOVE, and its quick action ſeem to recommend it to our trial, on this occaſion. It affects the brain very powerfully; excites long continued ſickneſs and vomiting; and has been ſuppoſed to produce a copious flow of ſaliva *(k)*. The laſt effect may be promoted by mercurial unctions, from which, in a few inſtances, ſome benefit ſeems to have been derived.

THE propagation of local nervous irritation to the brain is manifeſt in certain caſes of epilepſy; and is obviated by tight ligatures. This fact ſeems to point out a ſimilar treatment of the hydrophobous patient, as ſoon as the part bitten ſhews any ſigns of infection. Whether exciſion may then be adviſable muſt be determined by its ſituation, and by circumſtances, about which the attending phyſician or ſurgeon can alone decide. Should the wound open, it may be dilated, and waſhed with tepid water; after which, the gaſtric juice may be again applied. It has been found highly ſerviceable in foul ulcers; and is quick in producing its effects. It ſweet-

(i) PROBABLY the efficacy of half drowning the patient, which practice is ſaid to have been ſucceſsful, in a few inſtances, muſt have ariſen from the counter impreſſion made on the nervous ſyſtem. *Vid.* Vanſwieten. Comment. vol. III. p. 559.

(k) See Withering on the Fox-glove, p. 184.

ens

ens their fœtor; eaſes lancinating pains; and correcťs even the cancerous acrimony. Over the dreſſings a fermenting cataplaſm may be laid, compoſed of flour, honey, water, and yeaſt.

Such are the additions to your mean of prevention, and ſuch the curative plan, which I take the liberty of ſuggeſting to your conſideration. Both may perhaps ſeem ſuperfluous to you, whoſe generous zeal, for the good of your fellow-creatures, has elevated hope into confidence; and makes you ſay of the ſufferer, in the language of a well known amiable character, "he ſhall not die." I heartily wiſh that experience may fully confirm your ſanguine expectations. But, though I highly approve of your propoſal, as judiciouſly conceived; bidding fair to be ſucceſsful; and ſo eaſily practicable, that it ſhould be adopted, after the bite of every animal, to obviate even unſuſpected danger; yet, at preſent, I can regard it only as a rational hypotheſis, on a ſubject ſtill remaining in much obſcurity. We are ignorant of the peculiar properties of the canine *virus*; of the mode of its communication; and the parts of the animal ſyſtem affected by it. Are we then qualified to advance one ſtep beyond conjecture; and ought we to reſt ſatisfied with mere ablution, when it is uncertain what time is required for the agency of the deadly poiſon; and whether its baneful

baneful operation may not be accomplifhed, even before the completion of the fpeedy procefs you have pointed out? But admitting, what I fincerely hope may be found to be the truth, that the plentiful affufion of water will prove an effectual mean of prevention, there will ftill remain the neceffity of a curative plan, in thofe cafes, wherein the former has been neglected, or in which the difeafe has unexpectedly occurred.

I SHALL think myfelf happy, if the hints, I have propofed, merit your approbation: But it will render me ftill more happy, if they incite you to extend your refearches, and afford aid to your enlightened mind, in perfecting its difcoveries, on the important object of your inveftigation. *Fungar vice cotis—non inani munere.*

POSTSCRIPT.

Auguft 11, 1789. BEFORE this paper was fent to the prefs, I had not perufed the valuable OBSERVATIONS on the CAUSE and CURE of the TETANUS, by Dr. RUSH of PHILADELPHIA. He has obligingly fent me the volume of MEDICAL INQUIRIES, in which they are contained: And in the Appendix to his Effay, I am much pleafed to find a coincidence, in our ideas of the analogy between *Tetanus* and *Hydrophobia.*

phobia. I ſhall tranſcribe the paſſages, which have a reference to it.

" THE more I have conſidered the cauſes and " ſymptoms of *Hydrophobia*, the more I am " diſpoſed to aſcribe it to the ſame proximate " cauſe, as the *Tetanus.* 1. They both affect " the muſcles of deglutition. I have lately ſeen " a *Tetanus* brought on by a fractured leg, in " which an attempt to ſwallow the ſmalleſt " quantity of liquid, produced the ſame ſudden " and general convulſions which occur in the " *Hydrophobia.* 2. They both proceed from " cauſes which appear to be related to each " other, viz. from wounds, and from the action " of cold, after the body has been previouſly " weakened by heat and exerciſe. 3. They " both ſometimes appear as ſymptoms of the " ſame idiopathic diſorder, viz. the *Hyſteria.* " 4. They both yield to the ſame remedies, viz. " to the excitement of an inflammation in the " wounded part of the body, or to a long con- " tinued diſcharge of matter from it, and to " mercury."

" IF more facts ſhould occur, which ſhall " ſhew the relation that the *Tetanus* and *Hydro-* " *phobia* have to each other, perhaps we may " be led to conclude, that the wound, inflicted " by the teeth of a dog, ſometimes acts in the " ſame manner, in producing *Hydrophobia,* that " wounds made by a nail, or any other lacera-

" ting

"ting inſtrument act, in producing *Tetanus*; and "that both diſeaſes may be prevented or cured, "with equal certainty, by the ſame tonic reme-"dies."

THE *Tetanus* is aſcribed by Dr. Ruſh, to relaxation: And in the cure of it, he ſays, it is neceſſary not only to reſtore the ordinary tone of the ſyſtem, but to produce ſomething like the inflammatory *diatheſis*. A ſplinter under the nail, he affirms, produces no convulſions, if pain, inflammation, or ſuppuration follow the accident; and that the ſpirit of turpentine acts, by the excitement of pain and inflammation, in all wounds and fractures of tendinous parts. He has never known a ſingle inſtance of *Tetanus* from a wound, to which this remedy had been applied in time. In the iſland of St. Croix, the Negroes, he relates, always apply a plaſter, made of equal parts of ſalt and tallow, to their freſh wounds, to prevent the locked jaw: And that the ſalt never fails to produce ſome degree of inflammation.

THESE facts confirm the propriety of applying the gaſtric juice, to the part bitten by a ſuppoſed rabid animal, becauſe it is powerfully ſtimulant, as well as penetrating, ſolvent, and detergent. And if rennet be ſubſtituted, as recommended in page 374, there will be no neceſſity for ſeparating any more of the ſalt, than what adheres to it ſuperficially.

ESSAY

ESSAY XI.

MISCELLANEOUS

FACTS AND OBSERVATIONS:

ADDRESSED TO DOCTOR SIMMONS *(a)*.

THE great Lord Verulam recommends the collection of facts, experiments, and observations, as the best method of promoting the improvement of physic; and, in his essays, he expressly confines himself to "certain brief notes set down rather significantly than curiously." This mode of writing is consonant to the plan of the Medical Journal; and is often more agreeable to men of letters, than long and systematic compositions: For it precludes the labour of reading or of repeating elementary propositions, and well known truths; renders the detection of error more easy; facilitates the communication of new discoveries; and presents to the mind, in separate and distinct views, the real additions which

(a) Inserted in the London Medical Journal, vol. IV. p. 57.

which are made to ſcience (*b*). How far the influence of theſe conſiderations, or the ſanction of the high authority, I have quoted, may juſtify the following miſcellaneous remarks, I ſhall leave to your deciſion.

I. Retrograde Motion *of the* Lymphatics.

A very ingenious young phyſician and philoſopher, who, had he lived, would have done honour to his profeſſion, has advanced a variety of arguments to evince a nearer communication between the alimentary canal and the bladder, than by the ſanguiferous circulation (*c*). The following caſes may, perhaps, illuſtrate and confirm this doctrine.

Mrs. W. had laboured under a *diarrhœa* many weeks, when I was called to her aſſiſtance on the 13th of June 1780. I directed for her the following pills:

℞. *Extract. ligni Campech. gr. v.*
Philon. Londinenſ. gr. x.
Pulv. ipecac. gr. j.
Syrup. Cydon. q. ſ.
M. f. pil. iij. ter die ſumendæ.

By the uſe of theſe pills her diſorder ſoon abated.

(*b*) See the Preface to Part II.

(*c*) See Darwin's, Experiments, &c. Litchfield, printed 1780.

June

June 30th. She complained of nauſea, heat, and thirſt. The pulſe was not increaſed in velocity, and ſhe was ſtill inclined to be lax. The following mixture was preſcribed:

> ℞. *Aq. cinnam. ten.* ℥ *vij.*
> *Extract. ligni Campech.* ʒ *j.*
> *Sal. tart.* ℈ *iv.*
> *Syrup. Cydon.* ʒ *iij.*
> *M. cap.* ℥ *jſs. ter die in effervеſcentia, cum cochleare amplo ſucci limonum.*

This remedy ſeemed to obviate all her complaints. But in the morning of July the fifth, ſhe had a ſudden and urgent call to diſcharge her urine; and after voiding treble the uſual quantity, ſhe obſerved, that it was of a pink colour, inclining to purple, very ſimilar to that of the medicine which ſhe had taken. I found her under ſome alarm on account of this circumſtance; and examining her water in a glaſs, I was ſatisfied that its hue was different from that of blood: And from the appearance I concluded, that it was ſtrongly tinctured with logwood. In this opinion I was afterwards confirmed by its taſte, which was ſweetiſh and ſub-aſtringent; and by the deep purple it aſſumed, when a ſmall portion of the ſalt of ſteel was added to it. The urine of this patient had not, during the previous courſe of her illneſs, varied from its natural colour, although eight ſcruples of the *extractum ligni Campechenſis* had been adminiſtered. About an hour before the preſent ſingular evacuation, ſhe had taken the uſual doſe of her medicine; yet in the evening of the ſame day, her urine exhibited no marks of the logwood.

In this caſe there appears to have been a ſudden and copious tranſlation of urine into the bladder, probably by means of the retrograde motion of the lymphatics: And the fluids, conveyed with the lacteals, were ſtrongly imbued with a medicine, which, together with its colouring particles, evidently retained alſo its aſtringent quality *(d)*.

September 27th, 1780. Mrs. C. had been ill, more than two months, of a pulmonary conſumption, which was accompanied both with colliquative ſweats and a *diarrhœa*, when I was conſulted by her. I preſcribed a gentle emetic, and afterwards the following draughts:

R. *Emulſ. commun.* ℥*j.*
Myrrh. mucilag. gum. arab. ſolut. gr. xij.
Elix. pareg.

(d) Dr. Lewis, in his excellent *Materia Medica*, has obſerved, that logwood ſometimes colours the urine; but he does not ſeem to have been apprized, that it communicates aſtringency to it.

Sp. nit

Sp. nit dulc. aa. ℨ*ſs.*
Sal. tart. ℈*j.*
Extract. ligni Campech. gr. xv.
Succi limonum. ℥*ſs.*
M. f. hauſt. ter die in effervеſcentia ſumendus.

Her cough was alleviated, and the ſweating and *diarrhœa* almoſt entirely reſtrained by theſe draughts. But during the uſe of them, all the urine, which ſhe voided, had the colour of a dilute ſolution of logwood.

October 3d. The *diarrhœa* returned, and I had again recourſe to *extractum ligni Campechenſis*, which was now given every fourth hour, in doſes of fifteen grains, diſſolved in ſimple cinnamon water. The purging was ſoon checked, and the urine aſſumed the ſame pinky colour as before. A portion of it was turned black, by immerſing in it the blade of a table knife: Nor did the excretion change its appearance till the extract of logwood was laid aſide.

This inſtance of the *uniform* and *permanent* conveyance of a colouring aſtrictive matter to the bladder, may perhaps ſeem leſs favourable to the doctrine of a retrograde motion of the lymphatics, than the caſe before recited. But is it probable that ſo large a quantity of logwood, retaining its peculiar and active properties, could

 have

have been introduced into the blood veſſels, without occaſioning ſome unuſual ſymptoms? Or could the urine, in ſo ſhort a ſpace of time, have been replete with it, if it had been previouſly mixed with the whole maſs of circulating fluids? Be this, however, as it may, it is a curious and intereſting fact, that a vegetable aſtringent is capable of ſurmounting the powers of digeſtion, of paſſing into the abſorbent veſſels, and of being carried unchanged to the urinary organs. Various practical uſes may poſſibly be founded upon it; and it may furniſh a juſter theory of the action of the Peruvian bark, in glandular tumors, and diſorders of the lymphatic ſyſtem. Certain it is, that this very efficacious medicine is remarkably retentive of its virtues. Fuller ſays, with ſome degree of admiration, *Cum olim, experimenti cauſa, ejuſdem (corticis) decoxiſſem, non eo uſque vires ejus exhaurire valui, quin vel octavum decoctum adhuc amaricaret.* If his patience had permitted him to extend the experiment, he would have found, as I have done, that even twenty-five coctions, and thirty cold macerations, are inſufficient to exhauſt its virtues.

It is well known, that madder, taken internally, tinges the urine red; and that it produces a ſimilar effect even upon the bones of animals, though neither the fleſhy nor cartilaginous parts of the body ſuffer any alteration by its

its uſe. Nor will the bones, when thus ſtained, yield any colour to water, or ſpirit of wine. The root of this vegetable has a bitteriſh, and ſomewhat auſtere taſte; but I have not yet aſcertained, by any experiment, whether it impregnates the urine with an aſtrictive quality. The colouring matter of rhubarb is ſpeedily conveyed to the bladder; but the water thus imbued did not, in a late trial, exhibit the ſlighteſt appearance of purple, on mixing with it a ſmall quantity of the ſalt of ſteel.

Little attention has hitherto been paid to the change of quality produced, by food or medicine, on the ſecretions and excretions of the human body, although very uſeful information might be derived from it. Thus for example, could we medicate the milk of nurſes, we ſhould be better qualified to cure the diſeaſes of the children whom they ſuckle. There is a ſpecies of fœtid breath *(dyſodia pulmonica)*, to which perſons of a narrow cheſt and ſcorbutic habit are peculiarly incident. It ſeems to originate from the want of power to make a full expiration, by which too much perſpirable matter is retained, and corrupted by ſtagnation in the veſicles of the lungs. In ſuch caſes, I have found the moſt ſalutary effects from the uſe of myrrh and fixed air, internally adminiſtered. Theſe ſweetening and antiſeptic ſubſtances are

 probably

probably carried to the lungs, and difcharged together with the offenfive vapour, which they correct, at the fame time that they invigorate the fmalleft ramifications of the bronchiæ. For I cannot impute their action, *folely* at leaft, to their corroborant powers; becaufe neither fteel, the Peruvian bark, nor other tonics, are exhibited with the fame fuccefs.

It has been fhewn above, that an aftringent fubftance may be conveyed to the bladder, fo as ftrongly to impregnate the urine. And there is no reafon to prefume, that this is owing to any particular fubtlety in the *lignum Campechenfe.* Were proper tefts to be applied, the prefence of other remedies might, perhaps, be frequently difcovered in that recrementitious fluid. And thus we fhould have at command various means of cure, adapted to the diforders of thofe organs.

I shall clofe this fection with a paffage from Dr. Fuller, which, if it be the refult of accurate obfervation, corroborates what has been above advanced. Speaking of the balfam of Copaiba, he fays, *Sapore donatur amaro, acre, terebinthinaceo, admodum penetranti, et in ore durabili; atque licet videatur effe quædam terebinthinæ fpecies, urinam tamen odore violaceo minimè inficit; illam vero fapore amaro imbuit, ejufque et feri fanguinis, et falivæ muriaticam falfedinem mirifice delet.*

II. Reciprocal

II. Reciprocal Sympathy *between the* Stomach *and the* Lungs.

A gentleman, afflicted with a purulent expectoration, has found, by repeated experience, that his fits of coughing may often be suppreſſed by a draught of cold water, or a ſmall glaſs of wine. His courſe of life has been intemperate; and theſe remedies, by diminiſhing the *atonia* of the ſtomach, and producing a grateful ſenſation in that organ, allay, for a while, the irritation which ſubſiſts in the lungs. In ſuch caſes of *phthiſis*, which frequently occur, the exhibition of nitre, or other cold debilitating medicines, tends to aggravate the diſeaſe, and to haſten its fatal termination. To patients, under theſe circumſtances, porter is generally a very agreeable and ſalutary beverage. It quenches thirſt; quiets the cough; checks the ſweating; and, if drank only in ſmall quantities at once, does not accelerate the pulſe, or augment the hectic fever.

Ann Ogden, aged ten years, was admitted an out-patient of the Mancheſter infirmary, and put under my care on the twenty-ſecond of November 1779. On the eighteenth ſhe had been attacked with a moſt pungent pain in the ſtomach. The ſucceeding day, a violent ſpaſmodic cough enſued,

enſued, and her ſtools were obſerved to be bloody. She was ſoon relieved by opiates, mild purgatives, and a ſoft demulcent diet: For the ſwallowing of a pin gave riſe to theſe complaints; and the progreſs of them clearly evinces the ſympathy, which the lungs have with the ſtomach. To this law of the animal œconomy, phyſicians and phyſiologiſts have paid ſome attention; but they have not equally noticed the converſe of it; though it is no leſs certain, that various pulmonic affections may powerfully influence the ſtate of the ſtomach; and that the conſequent ſymptoms furniſh very important indications of cure.

A PHYSICIAN conſulted me, in February 1780, on account of a ſevere aſthma, of the humoral kind, to which he was ſubject. At the commencement of the diſeaſe, he could take ſeveral drachms of the *vinum ipecacoanhæ*. But as his diſorder increaſed, the irritability of his ſtomach became ſo great, that fifteen drops of the ſame wine often acted as an emetic. The medicine affording conſiderable eaſe to his breathing, he gradually augmented the doſe of it as he grew better, till he could bear a drachm or two without retching, and almoſt without nauſea.

MR. ——, in a ſevere peripneumony, took, every fourth hour, two ounces of a decoction of ſeneka

ſeneka root and liquorice (*e*). The remedy created no uneaſineſs, and ſeemed to give relief, whilſt the patient was in an erect poſture; but when he lay down, a poſition which rendered his breathing more difficult, every doſe of it aggravated the *dyſpnœa*. In this inſtance there ſeems to have been a reciprocal, or interchangeable action between the organs of digeſtion and of reſpiration. The increaſe of *dyſpnœa* produced an increaſe of irritability in the ſtomach; and the ſeneka root, under theſe circumſtances, proved ſo ſtimulant as to aggravate the oppreſſion of the lungs. This caſe, and I could cite many others, affords a ſtrong confirmation of the propriety of Sydenham's practice, in keeping his peripneumonic and pleuritic patients out of bed, as much as their ſtrength would permit.

III. Dysury.

Mr. —— of Knutsford, applied to me in January 1782, for advice concerning an arthritic vertigo. I directed a bliſter to the nape of his neck, and the following pills:

(*e*) The diſagreeable ſenſation, produced by the ſeneka root, in the fauces, is much abated by combining with it, in decoction, a ſufficient quantity either of the root, or the extract of liquorice, the demulcent quality of which is an excellent auxiliary in the peripneumony.

R. *Gum. guaiac.* ℨ *ij.*
Sal. ammon. vol. ℨ *j.*
Balſam guaiac. q. ſ.
M. f. pil. medioc. cap. iij. ter de die.

A violent ſtrangury enſued. The medicine was diſcontinued; the bliſter removed; and this painful complaint ſoon ceaſed. In a few days the pills were repeated; but the firſt doſe renewed the affection of the urinary organs. A drachm of the *ſpecies aromaticæ* was then ſubſtituted in lieu of the volatile ſalt; and this *formula* occaſioned no pain or inconvenience. But having more confidence in the efficacy of the pills firſt preſcribed, I adviſed the further trial of them at the end of ten days: They produced, however, a third time, the ſymptoms of ſtrangury, and were therefore entirely laid aſide. Is it not probable, that, in this caſe, there was a tranſlation of the gouty affection to the urinary paſſages, produced by the bliſter, and augmented by the ſtimulus of the volatile alkali? A prediſpoſition being thus formed in thoſe parts, the volatile ſalt alone might prove, afterwards, ſufficient to renew the malady.

There is a ſpecies of chronic DYSURY, to which perſons of an arthritic or ſcorbutic habit, and who have paſſed the meridian of life, are peculiarly incident. It is often miſtaken for the ſtone,

ſtone, and aggravated by the uſe of lithontriptics. Indeed it has many ſymptoms in common with that diſorder; ſuch as frequent and urgent calls to make water; pain at each extremity of the *urethra*; a mucous diſcharge; *teneſmus*; and ſometimes a ſuppreſſion of urine. But the patients, who labour under it, feel no uneaſy weight in the *peritonæum*, and always void their water with much leſs difficulty, in an erect, than in an horizontal poſture. The complaint, alſo, may be further diſtinguiſhed from the ſtone by having ſhorter intervals of eaſe; by more frequently injuring the retentive power of the bladder, and by occaſioning no ſudden interruption to the ſtream of urine, in the abſence of pain. It ſeems to ariſe from an acrid defluxion on the internal coat of the bladder, which is thereby rendered ſo exquiſitely ſenſible, that the ſtimulus of the urine becomes almoſt intolerable; and very frequent efforts are excited to expel it. Theſe efforts, however, ſhould be reſtrained, becauſe they tend to increaſe the pain and irritation of the bladder, and to prevent the complete diſcharge of its contents; for that organ cannot effectually contract itſelf without a due degree of previous diſtenſion.

I HAVE tried various remedies in this diſorder, but have found none ſo ſucceſsful as mercury, which ſeldom fails to afford relief, and generally

produces

produces a cure, if adminiſtered with perſeverance, and in ſufficient quantity. According to the urgency of the caſe, one, two, or three ſcruples of the *unguentum cœruleum fortius* ſhould be rubbed into the thighs every night, till a ſlight ptyaliſm enſues: The ſymptoms for the moſt part abate, before the ſpitting comes on, and after it has continued a while, they diſappear entirely.

I WAS firſt induced to adopt this mode of treatment, from my experience of the ſalutary operation of the remedy, recommended by Dr. Gilchriſt, in a diſorder of the bladder, which bears ſome analogy to that which I have deſcribed *(f)*; but having found that the mercurial pill is apt to diſturb the bowels, and conſequently that it is leſs certain of admiſſion into the ſyſtem, I have, in my later practice, preferred the uſe of the *unguentum cœruleum*. In ſlighter caſes, indeed, I ſometimes give half a grain of calomel, with two grains of James's fever powder, twice every day; and this ſmall doſe of mercury, if duly continued, may ſuffice to effect a cure, without producing any ſalivation, or even ſoreneſs of the mouth. In a late inſtance, an habitual head-ach, with which a difficulty and pain in making water were complicated, gave way to this remedy.

(f) Phyſical and Literary Eſſays, vol. III.

From

From the ſalutary operation of mercury in the dyſury, it may be ſuſpected, perhaps, that the diſeaſe originated from the *lues venerea.* I formerly entertained this idea myſelf; but further experience has convinced me, that it has no foundation in more than half the caſes which occur; and conſequently, in explaining the action of the remedy preſcribed, we muſt not have recourſe to the ſecret powers of a ſpecific or an antidote.

MANCHESTER, FEB. 26, 1783.

ESSAY XII.

MISCELLANEOUS

PRACTICAL OBSERVATIONS;

COMMUNICATED TO DOCTOR DUNCAN *(a)*.

FLOWERS OF ZINC.

SEVERAL years ago I was consulted by a young gentleman, about nineteen years of age, who laboured under a deep cough, attended with a hoarseness. He was returning from Liverpool, the place of his apprenticeship, to pass some time with his friends in the eastern part of this county. I recommended a milk diet, gentle exercise, country air, and a decoction of the seneka root and liquorice. How long he pursued this plan I am uncertain, as I never saw him afterwards. But my friend Dr. Dobson informed me that he came back to Liverpool, and was put under his care. Dr.

(a) Inserted in the Medical Commentaries, vol. V. p. 166.

Alcock

Alcock was alſo called to his aſſiſtance, and many judicious remedies were preſcribed, but with no laſting good effect. Dr. Dobſon now began to ſuſpect that his cough was ſpaſmodic, and directed for him the flowers of zinc. This remedy, in a few weeks, produced a perfect cure; and the young gentleman has ever ſince, I believe, remained free from his diſorder. The communication of this account firſt induced me to make trial of zinc, in various pulmonary affections; and I ſhall relate a few inſtances of the ſucceſs, which has attended the exhibition of this remedy.

Mrs. P. aged twenty-eight, a lady whoſe conſtitution had been much impaired by frequent child-bearing, was attacked with a ſevere aſthma, of the nervous kind, in the winter of the year 1776. The aſthma was cured by the uſual methods of treatment; but left behind it a deep convulſive cough, the ſucculſions of which were no leſs frequent than violent. *Gum ammoniac, paregoric elixir, ſp. nitri dulcis,* and other remedies, were ſucceſſively tried. Little or no relief being obtained, I had recourſe to the flowers of zinc, beginning with half a grain twice in the day, and gradually increaſing the doſe to a grain and a half. The beneficial effects of this antiſpaſmodic were ſoon viſible; and in eight or ten days the patient was freed from her cough. A

 relapſe

relapſe afterwards occurred from cold. The ſame medicine was repeated, and the cough again yielded to it as before.

T. B. P. a youth about ten years of age, had a deep hoarſe cough, without any expectoration. The ſound of it was very unuſual, and not to be deſcribed; and it was attended with a quick, but feeble pulſe, fluſhings in the face, and pain in the breaſt. Every morning, about two o'clock, the cough recurred with great violence, and continued, almoſt without intermiſſion, till four or five. There was reaſon to ſuſpect worms, and I had been careful to cleanſe the *primæ viæ*, on the firſt attack of the diſorder. A ſolution of ſpermaceti and gum ammoniac, with a few drops of *tinct. thebaic.* having no effect, I had recourſe to the flowers of zinc. Half a grain was given at noon, and the ſame doſe repeated at bed-time. The night paſſed with only a ſlight return of the cough; and, by continuing the uſe of this remedy, the youth perfectly recovered in a few days.

Mrs. B. laboured under a *phthiſis pulmonalis*, during the whole period of pregnancy. The violence of her cough occaſioned a premature delivery; and continued after that event, without abatement. Opiates never failed to afford relief; but they ſometimes affected her head ſo much, that ſhe intreated me to try ſome other remedy. She

She was of an irritable habit, and was troubled with ſpaſmodic pains, in various parts of her body. I preſcribed the flowers of zinc; which ſoon mitigated her cough, and eaſed her wandering pains. This medicine was continued only two days; but the cough remained moderate, more than double that ſpace of time. It recurred, however, with ſeverity, and I had again recourſe to the zinc. The beneficial effects of this remedy were not now ſo great, or ſo immediate as before; but they were ſufficiently apparent to encourage perſeverance in the uſe of it. In a few days, a truce from the violence of the cough was again obtained; and the patient was enabled to diſcharge great quantities of phlegm with facility, and without pain; for her expectoration was always moſt free and copious, when the cough was gentle and moderate. This evacuation, with the hectic fever which accompanied it, gradually waſted her fleſh and ſtrength; and there was no further occaſion for a repetition of the flowers of zinc: For, in the laſt ſtage of a pulmonary conſumption, it often happens, that the ſymptoms of the diſorder, by degrees, grow leſs painful and violent, as the patient approaches nearer and nearer to the termination of life. I have known the pulſe to ſink gradually from one hundred and thirty to ſeventy ſtrokes in a minute, and to continue about this number during ten or twelve days preceding death. Nor will this fact seem wonderful, when we reflect, that the functions of the brain are no less injured by inanition, than by plenitude; and, that the sensibility and irritability of the heart and blood vessels must be regulated by, and dependent upon the state of the nervous system *(b)*.

COLIC.

(b) August 1, 1789. ZINC is a very useful remedy in the HOOPING COUGH, administered twice or thrice daily, in nauseating doses.

IN cases of great debility of the stomach, when too large a proportion of mucus is secreted, zinc may be given with great advantage, and repeated occasionally, as an emetic. The operation is generally speedy, easy, and succeeded by a sensible increase of tone in the digestive organs.

I LATELY prescribed for —— B. Esq. on account of a chronic *dyspnœa*, pills composed of myrrh, zinc, and camphor. The dose of zinc, daily given, was at first only three, but afterwards six grains. About the beginning of July, I was informed that "the patient had been alarmed with a disagreeable "sensation in the whole of one side, an inability, as it were, "at times to use either the leg or the arm; and that he sometimes felt a similar affection in the tongue, when talking, "which momentarily deprived him of the power of articulation."

IN consequence of this account, *sal martis* was substituted for the zinc; and the patient experienced no longer the symptoms described. There is some presumption, therefore, that they were owing to the action of this medicine. Yet I have administered it, during a long space of time, to very delicate and

COLIC.

In violent colics, attended with vomiting and an obſtinate conſtipation of the bowels, it has been the common practice amongſt phyſicians to give opiates in conjunction with purgatives. This method of treatment has been lately improved, by adminiſtering the opiate firſt, and the purgative an hour or two afterwards. But I take the liberty of ſuggeſting to you another mode, which, as far as my own experience extends, has proved the moſt ſucceſsful. I direct three or four ounces of a ſtrong decoction of poppy heads, with twenty, thirty, or forty drops of *tinctura thebaica*, to be injected into the inteſtines, and retained as long as poſſible. If it be ſpeedily diſcharged, the clyſter is repeated till the pain is relieved, and the vomiting ceaſes. A doſe of calomel and jalap, or of any other briſk cathartic, is then adminiſtered; and its operation quickened by the uſe of ſenna tea, of a ſolution of the neutral ſalts, or of

and irritable ſubjects, without ever before obſerving from it any injurious effects. Dr. Cullen, however, quotes the Experiments of M. Hellot, as affording a proof that zinc, in a certain quantity, may operate as a violent poiſon (Mat. Med. vol. II. p. 30.). I fear it ſometimes contains a mixture of arſenic: Particular care, therefore, ſhould be employed in the preparation of it; nor ſhould it ever be long adminiſtered in large doſes.

caſtor oil. By this proceſs, evacuations are procured with more eaſe, certainty, and expedition, than by any other which I have tried. For opium, when given in a clyſter, does not check the periſtaltic motion of the inteſtines, nor counteract the operation of any purgative, ſo powerfully, as when received into the ſtomach. And, in this way, it is moſt efficacious in alleviating the ſickneſs, and in putting a ſtop to the violent retchings with which colics are often attended. The taſte of laudanum is ſo nauſeous, that it is often rejected as ſoon as ſwallowed. And, if the *extractum thebaicum* be given in a ſolid form, time muſt be allowed for its ſolution, before any effect can be expected from it.

HYDROCEPHALUS INTERNUS.

The fatality of the *hydrocephalus internus* has been acknowledged, and lamented by the moſt experienced and intelligent phyſicians. The late Dr. Whytt, of Edinburgh, has recorded twenty caſes, which baffled his ſkill and judgment; and a phyſician of the higheſt reputation, in his excellent remarks on this diſorder, candidly confeſſes, that it is not in his power to ſuggeſt any probable means of curing it, and that it has hitherto diſappointed all his attempts, both when confided in alone, and in conſultation with the ableſt of the faculty *(a)*.

(c) See Medical Obſervations and Inquiries, vol. V. p. 40.

About ſix weeks ago, the ſame very ingenious friend, whom I mentioned to you under the article of zinc, acquainted me, that he had successfully adminiſtered mercury, in ſuch quantity as to ſalivate, in one inſtance of the *hydrocephalus internus*. As the caſe appeared to be clear and indubitable, and the efficacy of the remedy ſufficiently probable, I determined to avail myſelf of ſo important a diſcovery, on the firſt occurrence of the diſeaſe in my circle of practice. This has lately happened, and I ſhall give you a minute hiſtory of it, copied *verbatim* from my regiſter.

September 4, 1777. Master H. a child at the breaſt, aged ſeven months, has laboured about a fortnight under a ſlow irregular fever. His eyes have been now and then a little diſtorted; he has been affected with ſome degree of ſtupor; his gums have been inflamed and tender; and his mouth uncommonly dry. No tooth has yet made its appearance. An emetic has been adminiſtered; a bliſter applied to his back; and his belly has been kept ſoluble by repeated ſmall doſes of magneſia. During the action of the bliſter, he was thought to be much better; but he ſoon relapſed into his former ſtate.

About three o'clock this morning, he was convulſed; at nine I ſaw him, and, from his countenance, inſtantly ſuſpected a dropſy of the brain. The ſymptoms confirmed my apprehenſions. His ſkin was hot, yet his pulſe beat only ſeventy-eight ſtrokes in a minute, which were irregular. The pupils of his eyes were conſiderably, but unequally dilated; nor did they contract much, when a lighted candle was ſuddenly held before them. He often ſquinted, eſpecially with the right eye, and ſeemed to take no notice of any object around him. He refuſed the breaſt, and ſeldom ſwallowed, till the lips and tongue had been ſtimulated with a feather. During ſeveral days paſt, he had been frequently obſerved to rub the end of his noſe, when his hand was at liberty. And, notwithſtanding his ſtupor, he had been uncommonly watchful. I examined his head, and found a manifeſt tumor of the *bregma*, which had never before been noticed. Convinced, by all theſe circumſtances, that the child laboured under the *hydrocephalus internus*, and that he was now in the ſecond ſtage of that diſorder, I directed ten grains of the *unguentum mercuriale mitius* to be rubbed into his thighs, every three hours, till the mouth ſhould be affected; and a tea-ſpoonful of the following mixture to be given, whenever the convulſive ſymptoms recurred.

℞. *Salis ammon. vol.* ℈*i. Succi Limon.* ℥*vi. Moſch. opt. mucilagine G. Arabic. ſolut. gr. vi. Sacch. alb. q. ſ. ad gratiam. M.*

SMALL

Small bliſters were applied on each ſide of the head, juſt below the *bregma*, and a folded rag, frequently moiſtened with brandy, was laid upon the tumor, to promote abſorption. An emetic had been given early in the morning, before I ſaw the child, by which a large quantity of bile was diſcharged; and a veſicatory had alſo been applied to his leg.

September 5th, nine o'clock. The child has had frequent convulſions in the night; his right eye is much diſtorted; and it has been remarked, that he ſeldom moves the right hand. The pulſe beats one hundred and twenty ſtrokes in a minute. Two ſcruples of the mercurial ointment have been uſed, and he has taken five grains of muſk. A large diſcharge of ſerum has been produced by the bliſters. Five o'clock, P. M. The tumor of the head is ſenſibly diminiſhed; the child's mouth is now moiſt, and often filled with ſaliva; and his tongue appears to be ſwollen. His pulſe beats one hundred and forty-ſix ſtrokes in a minute. I directed another bliſter to be applied to the head.

September 6th. His convulſions have been much ſlighter; his eye is leſs frequently diſtorted; and the pupils of each are more contracted. The ſtupor is conſiderably abated; the child ſeems to take ſome notice, diſtinguiſhes taſtes, and ſwallows freely. The muſk has been continued;

continued; and half a drachm more of the mercurial ointment has been consumed. A clyster was injected last night, but ineffectually. I therefore prescribed a grain of jalap, mixed with an equal quantity of sugar, to be given every three hours till a motion to stool succeeded.

September 7th. THE child has passed the night more comfortably, but not free from convulsions. His head has sweated profusely; and the blisters have run much. The tumor of the *bregma* is considerably reduced. The jalap operated gently last night, and the mercurial unction has been twice repeated. There is an evident mitigation of all the symptoms.

September 8th. ABOUT eleven o'clock last night, the child was attacked with severe convulsions, which recurred frequently, till six o'clock this morning. He has had a short sleep, and is now composed. His pulse beats one hundred and forty strokes in a minute; his heat is moderate; and his skin soft and perspirable. The mercurial ointment has been again used; but, though his gums and tongue are sore and very moist, his breath is not offensive. I directed a grain of calomel to be immediately given, to procure a stool; and a blister to be applied to the *occiput*.

September 10th. A distant call from Manchester, prevented me from visiting the child yesterday.

yeſterday. He has paſſed two nights almoſt entirely free from convulſions. Ten grains of the mercurial ointment have been again rubbed into his thighs. The doſe of calomel occaſioned three very offenſive ſtools; and directions are given to repeat it, as he is again coſtive. The bliſter applied to the *occiput*, like the others, has produced a very copious diſcharge. The tumor of the head is now ſcarcely perceptible. Pulſe one hundred and twenty.

September 12th. At twelve o'clock laſt night, the convulſions recurred with greater violence than ever, and ſtill continue. Two teeth have almoſt protruded through the upper and the ſame number through the lower gum. Pulſe one hundred and ſixty, tremulous, and irregular. I directed that the child ſhould be immediately put into a warm bath, and that the following remedies ſhould be adminiſtered.

℞. *Infuſi. rad. Valer. fortiſſimi* ℥*ii.*
Aſſæfætid. electæ. ℈*ſs. M. f. Enema ſtatim injiciendum.*

℞. *Tinct Valer. volat.* ʒ*ii. Dentur guttæ jii. ſubindè è cochleari parvulo Infuſi rad. Valer. ſylv. ſub forma Theæ parati.*

The convulſions continued, but with leſs violence; and the child expired about one o'clock in the afternoon.

The

The deplorable cafe, which I have related, appears to have originated from the irregular action, produced in the fyftem, by dentition; and from the want of a due fecretion of faliva in the mouth, by which the fluid difcharges were probably increafed in the ventricles of the brain. That thefe difcharges were diminifhed, and that the extravafated water was abforbed by the powerful action of the mercury, may be prefumed from the mitigation of all the fymptoms which fucceeded the falivation. And, I am inclined to believe that the convulfions, under which the child expired, were more owing to the irritation of his gums, by the protrufion of four teeth, than to any remaining water in the brain: For the tumor of the head had entirely difappeared; and, after death, there was a manifeft depreffion of the *bregma*. During the fpace of a week, one hundred and ten grains of the *unguentum mercuriale mitius*, which contain about twenty-two grains of mercury, were confumed, in the ufual way of friction. Perhaps half of this quantity might be abforbed, and carried into the courfe of circulation; to which may be added, part of the two grains of calomel adminiftered internally. The fymptoms of the falivation were not violent; and the effects of the mercury did not appear formidable or alarming, even to the parents of the child, who were apprized of the nature

nature of the diſorder, and fully approved of the trial of this new method of treatment. The death of my patient will not, I hope, diſcourage the farther uſe of the remedy employed, when it is recollected, that he was in the moſt irritable period of infancy; that he was ſtruggling under dentition; and, that a dropſy of the brain was not ſuſpected till the concluſion of its ſecond ſtage, when the nervous ſyſtem had been ſhocked by ſevere convulſions.

EXTRACT OF A

SECOND LETTER TO DR. DUNCAN.

HYDROCEPHALUS INTERNUS(a).

THOUGH the arguments of your very ingenious correſpondent, Dr. Simmons, have not produced any change in my ſentiments; yet I think myſelf obliged by his candour, and honoured by his politeneſs. And as I am perſuaded that his ſtrictures proceed from the love of truth, and a ſpirit of benevolence, I doubt

(a) Inſerted in the Medical Commentaries, vol. VI. p. 224.

not

not it will afford him ſatisfaction to hear, that farther experience has furniſhed me with fuller evidence of the ſafety and efficacy of mercury, timely adminiſtered, in the *hydrocephalus internus*.

ONE of my own children, a girl, aged three years and three months, has lately been a ſevere ſufferer under this alarming malady. As ſoon as the characteriſtic ſymptoms of the diſeaſe clearly manifeſted themſelves, I laid aſide all other remedies, convinced, by repeated obſervation, of their inſufficiency; and truſted ſolely, though with much ſolicitude, to the internal and external uſe of mercury. In forty-eight hours, ſigns of amendment appeared, and her recovery was perfected in ſix days. During this ſpace of time, thirteen grains of calomel were adminiſtered, and ſeven ſcruples of the *unguentum mercuriale fortius* carefully rubbed into her legs.

I do not ſend you a detail of the caſe, becauſe I ſhall probably offer it myſelf to the public. For, having marked every circumſtance of the diſeaſe with the watchful and anxious attention of a parent, I may, perhaps, have acquired a more intimate knowledge of its nature, and of the peculiar operation of mercury in the cure of it, than can be obtained in the ordinary courſe of a phyſician's practice. I am willing to hope,

at

at leaſt, that I have been able to guard againſt deception.

In the treatment of the *hydrocephalus internus*, no remedy has had a more general trial than bliſters: I have often employed them myſelf; but never yet ſaw any inſtance, in which they could be ſaid to produce other than palliative effects. The publication of Dr. Ambroſe Dawſon, referred to in the laſt N°. of the Medical Commentaries, has not yet fallen into my hands; but that learned and judicious phyſician informs me, that his notes were not ſufficiently minute and particular, to aſcertain the caſes to be of the malady in queſtion. The fatality of the diſorder, he ſays, convinced him that purgatives and diuretics are given on a bad theory; and the main deſign of his paper is to incite the faculty, to attempt the diſcovery of a more ſucceſsful method of cure.

Mention is made of only one bliſter, in the curious hiſtory of a dropſy of the brain, communicated ſome time ago, by my friend Dr. Dobſon. This was applied between the ſhoulders, on the fourteenth of February 1775. On the fifteenth, the diſeaſe ſeems, by the doctor's letter which now lies before me, to have made a rapid progreſs; the mercurial courſe was therefore commenced, and continued till the twenty-ſecond, when the child was out of danger.

ESSAY XIII.

AN ACCOUNT

OF AN

EARTHQUAKE IN SEPTEMBER 1777(a).

ON Sunday, the fourteenth of September, at eleven o'clock in the forenoon, a ſevere ſhock of an earthquake was felt at Mancheſter, which extended itſelf through a circuit of more than three hundred miles. The morning was unclouded and ſerene, the wind was eaſterly, but ſuddenly veered into the oppoſite quarter, about the time of the earthquake; and the air was temperately warm, without any ſulphureous, or other offenſive vapours.

THE ſummer has been cold and wet; but towards the end of Auguſt, the weather changed, and has continued dry and pleaſant, with few intermiſſions to the preſent time, September 26,

(a) Inſerted in the Annual Regiſter, vol XX. p. 78.

1777.

1777. The Aurora Borealis has not often appeared, and ſtorms of thunder and lightning have been uncommonly rare. Two months ago, a water ſpout is ſaid to have fallen near Huddersfield, a town in Yorkſhire, between twenty and thirty miles diſtant from Mancheſter.

DURING the ſpace of three weeks before the earthquake, vegetation was uncommonly vigorous. On the Sunday preceding it, an electrical machine collected more fire that it had ever been known to do before.

DIFFERENT churches in this town ſeem to have been very differently affected by the ſhock. St. John's church was moſt, St. Paul's leaſt agitated. The former is built of ſtone upon a dry rocky foundation; and the galleries are ſupported with pillars of caſt iron. The latter is a brick building; has a clayey wet foundation, and a common ſewer runs under it. Four leaden ſpouts alſo, which convey rain from the roof, *appear* to paſs into the ground. I ſay *appear* to paſs, becauſe at the bottom they are covered with wood, and the clergyman of the church has not yet aſcertained the fact.

THE bell of St. Mary's church was heard to ring during the ſhock. An electrical rod paſſes through the ſteeple, which may perhaps account for this peculiarity.

The shock was trifling at my country house at Hart-Hill, which has many high trees about it; whereas it was severely felt at a gentleman's house in the neighbourhood not so circumstanced.

A noise was antecedent to the concussion, and gave the alarm to many persons, who were insensible of the shock. It was particularly loud in several houses which have electrical conductors.

Few travellers, either on horseback or in carriages, perceived the earthquake. The passage boat upon the Duke of Bridgewater's canal was stopped in its course, as if it had struck upon a cable, or other obstacle. Many persons seemed to be electrified by the shock; and wandering rheumatic pains succeeded it.

A lady received a sudden stroke on her head, during the earthquake. She was standing in a closet, on the outside wall of which, opposite to her head, a leaden spout terminated, so as to form an imperfect conductor.

I am informed by a gentleman, whose cattle graze in a large pasture near his house, that he observed them to be exceedingly agitated before the earthquake; and that previous to it, they all ran to their usual place of shelter in storms.

These facts cannot be explained by any supposition of fermentations or explosions in the bowels of the earth, unless they be considered as agents

agents in the production and accumulation of the electrical fluid: And many of them seem to confirm the theory of Dr. Stukeley and Signor Beccaria, concerning earthquakes. But in whatever manner such awful and tremendous events may be accounted for, the pious philosopher, when he contemplates them, extends his views beyond all secondary causes; and directing them to the great Author of the universe, regards the laws of nature only as the exertions of his divine energy.

*** My friend Dr. Priestley, to whom I have communicated the preceding observations, and who is much better acquainted with electricity than I am, seems to be fully satisfied that the late earthquake is not to be ascribed to any subterranean cause. And he is persuaded that he shall be able to produce similar phænomena, by means of a most powerful and magnificent electrical machine, now in the possession of Lord Shelburne, from which he has seen sparks taken in the open air, at the distance of twenty inches.

OBSERVATIONS ON THE

SILK COTTON OF SUMATRA(a).

A FEW weeks ago I received, from the Archbiſhop of York, a ſmall quantity of the *bombax ceiba*, or ſilk cotton of Sumatra, with a requeſt that I would inquire, whether it might not be applied to ſome important uſes, in the manufactures of Mancheſter. The ſpecimen was given to his Grace by Mr. William Marſden, F. R. S. late ſecretary to the preſident and council of Fort Marlborough, and author of a valuable work, entitled the Hiſtory of Sumatra. I have ſhewn the cotton to ſeveral of our moſt ingenious manufacturers, who unite in admiring its ſoftneſs, fineneſs, beauty, and ſilky gloſs; but are apprehenſive, from the ſhortneſs and extreme tenderneſs of its filaments, that it is unfit for the operations of carding, ſpinning, or weaving.

IT occurred to me that, in the manufacture of hats, no operation ſeems to be required, which would overſtrain the texture of this delicate ſubſtance;

(a) Inſerted in the New Ann. Regiſt. for 1787, p. [144.]

that

that it is adapted to the reception of a bright and permanent dye; and that its finenefs and foftnefs might render it a good fubftitute for beaver. A gentleman, however, converfant in this branch of trade, to whom I fhewed the cotton, and communicated the foregoing conjectures, is of opinion that it has not fufficient firmnefs for matting together, in the ftructure of a hat.

NOTWITHSTANDING thefe difcouragements, I am not yet convinced, that the Sumatra cotton might not, by a mixture with other fpecies, with filk, or with worfted, be rendered ufeful to our manufactures. And poffibly its fibres may, when feparately employed, be fufficiently ftrengthened for the wheel or the loom, by undergoing a due preparation. Hairs of the fame length vary much in their powers of extenfion, when wetted with different fluids, as Dr. Bryan Robinfon has proved *(b)*. And may we not infer, from analogy, that the fame diverfity would take place in the filaments of cotton? The fact might eafily be afcertained; and I take the liberty of recommending the inveftigation of it to fome ingenious experimenter, interefted in the improvement of our manufactures. In this undertaking three objects may be held in view: 1. To in-

(b) SEE his Treatife on the Virtues and Operations of Medicines, p. 178.

creaſe the powers of coheſion in the fibres of cotton, without proportionably augmenting their powers either of extenſion or elaſticity. 2. To augment the power of extenſion, without affecting that of elaſticity. 3. To increaſe the power of elaſticity, in conjunction with that of extenſion. Different ſubſtances may be found to poſſeſs qualities adapted to theſe ſeveral ends, each of which may be appropriate to ſome particular kind of manufacture.

SINCE the foregoing remarks were written, I have conſulted Mr. Marſden's Hiſtory of Sumatra, and ſhall tranſcribe from it, what he delivers concerning the *bombax ceiba.* "The ſilk cot-"ton is to be met with in every village. "This is, to appearance, one of the moſt beau-"tiful raw materials the hand of Nature has "preſented. Its fineneſs, gloſs, and delicate "ſoftneſs render it, to the ſight and touch, much "ſuperior to the labour of the ſilk worm; but, "owing to the ſhortneſs and brittleneſs of the "ſtaple, it is eſteemed unfit for the reel and "loom; and is only applied to the unworthy "purpoſes of ſtuffing pillows, and mattreſſes. "Poſſibly it has not undergone a fair trial in the "hands of our ingenious artiſts; and we may "yet ſee it converted into a valuable manufac-"ture. It grows in pods, from four to ſix "inches long, which burſt open when ripe. The

"ſeeds

"seeds entirely resemble black pepper; but are "without taste. The tree is remarkable from "the branches growing out perfectly straight "and horizontal, and being always three, form-"ing equal angles at the same height. The "diminutive shoots, likewise, grow flat; and the "several gradations of branches observe the same "regularity to the top. Some travellers have "called it the umbrella tree; but the piece of "furniture called a dumb waiter, exhibits a more "striking picture of it*(a)*."

ON THE

ACID OF TAR*(b)*.

TAR, boiled to dryness, without addition, yields an acid liquor, in considerable quantity, which the workmen injudiciously throw away; though an able chemist informs us, he has known a person in France save by it many thousand dollars*(c)*. I have lately procured several gallons of it, from a large pitch manufactory at Hull.

(a) History of Sumatra, p. 126.

(b) Inserted in the New Ann. Regist. for 1787, p. [145.]

(c) See Newman's Chemistry, by Lewis, p. 288.

Hull. It exceeds greatly in pungency other vegetable acids; and I am persuaded that it might be employed to advantage, both in pharmacy and the arts, as a cheap and active menstruum. Such are its corrosive powers, that, I am informed, it soon proves destructive to the large metallic vessels, in which it is distilled. If these be of copper, they bear about a year's working; if made of tin, they are presently eaten into holes, like a honey-comb. It is not easy to form an exact estimate of the comparative strength of different acids; but, from several experiments which I made, it appeared probable, that the acid of tar is to the *sp. vitriol. fort.* in this respect, as one to fourteen. For five drops of the former, and seventy drops of the latter gave the like degree of pungency to equal portions of water; and seemed to be saturated with equal quantities of fixed alkali. A thin piece of lead, weighing twenty-three grains, was suspended by a string, several weeks, in two ounces of the acid of tar. The menstruum gradually lost its natural hue, and assumed a light yellow. At first the colouring matter swam on the surface; but afterwards the whole fluid became uniformly transparent. Its acidity was diminished, and a slight degree of sweetness was perceptible in it. The piece of lead, when taken out, weighed only seventeen grains and a half; and the surface of it

was

was covered with a black pigment which ſtained the fingers.

ANOTHER piece of lead, exactly ſimilar in form and weight, was immerſed, during the ſame period of time, in two ounces of white wine vinegar, with the loſs only of half a grain.

FROM the reſult of theſe experiments I think we may conclude, that the acid of tar would be preferable to vinegar, both in the preparation of *ſaccharum ſaturni*, and *acetum lithargyrites*; perhaps if it could be freed, by farther diſtillation, from the pitchy matter which it contains, the manufacture of ceruſſe or white lead might be greatly benefited by it. For the pigment, communicated to the piece of lead ſuſpended in the acid of tar, probably aroſe from the ſuperabundant phlogiſton of the menſtruum. A ſimilar phænomenon occurs in the operation for making lunar cauſtic. The cryſtals of ſilver, when fuſed, aſſume a black colour, which Mr. Macquer aſcribes to the inflammable principle of the nitrous acid, that attaches itſelf ſuperficially to the ſilver. Perhaps the acid of tar might be employed, in a purified ſtate, for making verdigriſe. I attempted to aſcertain this point; but an accident put an end to my experiment, before it was completed.

As I have given ſpecimens of this acid to ſeveral of my chemical friends, I flatter myſelf that

that ſome valuable diſcoveries will be made of its application to pharmacy, and to the arts.

MAY 14, 1783.

SINCE this paper was written, I have been favoured with a letter from Mr. Charles Taylor, an eminent callico printer and a competent judge of the ſubject, who expreſſes himſelf in the following terms: "The acid of tar, I am confident, might be rendered of great conſequence "in various manufactures, particularly in the "callico printing buſineſs, in which a very great "conſumption is made of ſolutions of iron in the "vegetable acid, as well as of ſolutions of lead "in the ſame acid. I think the ſolution of lead "in the acid of tar, though the liquor may not "be perfectly clear, would be an excellent ſub"ſtitute for the *ſaccharum ſaturni*, uſed in that "branch of buſineſs; more particularly as the ex"pence of the cryſtallization would be avoided."

"THE acid liquor, which is procured from pit coal when diſtilled for tar, is at preſent thrown away, as I have been informed by a perſon who is much engaged in this buſineſs." See Biſhop Watſon's Chemical Eſſays, vol. II. p. 353.

OBSERVA-

OBSERVATIONS

ON THE CONSTRUCTION AND POLITY OF

PRISONS;

Communicated to the EDITOR of the GENT. MAGAZINE (a).

SIR, MANCHESTER, JUNE 22.

THE erection of a new gaol for the division of Ipswich, and of a house of correction for that of St. Edmond's-Bury, having engaged the attention of the inhabitants of Suffolk, Capel Lofft, Esq. an able and active magistrate of that county, consulted Dr. John Jebb concerning their polity and construction. The answer returned by him was printed in 1785; and I was honoured by Mr. Lofft with a copy of the tract, which is now inserted in the second vol. of the Doctor's works. It is written in the true spirit of philanthropy, and contains many judicious and important observations. But, differing in opinion from the amiable and respectable author on one essential point, I

(a) Inserted in the Gent. Mag. for Sept. 1787, p. 765.

availed

availed myſelf of the privilege granted me, and tranſmitted my ſentiments to Mr. Lofft without reſerve, truſting they would be communicated to Dr. Jebb, whoſe friendly correſpondence I ſometimes enjoyed. But the melancholy event of his death occurred about the time when my letter arrived; and it was delivered to Lord Chedworth, as chairman, for the conſideration of the juſtices at the quarter-ſeſſion. If you think ſuch a mite towards the general ſtock of public information, on a ſubject which now happily intereſts the phyſician, the philoſopher, and the ſtateſman, in almoſt every country of Europe, will be an acceptable contribution, the publication of it in your Repoſitory will oblige your conſtant reader.

Copy *of a* Letter *to* Capel Lofft, *Eſq. of* Troſton Hall, *near* Bury, *in* Suffolk, *on the Subject of* Prisons.

MANCHESTER, JAN. 26, 1786.

SIR,

PERMIT me to return my grateful acknowledgments for your very obliging letter; which, though dated September 22, 1785, arrived only three weeks ago, together with an intereſting Tract on the Conſtruction and Polity of Priſons.

I admire

I admire the ability, and honour the patriotic zeal, which this little work diſplays; and perhaps I ſhall but evince my reſpect for the editor, by offering to him ſuch comments and remarks as the peruſal of it has ſuggeſted to my mind.

Though under the form of a query, it ſeems to be laid down as a *poſtulatum*, that, when infection has once taken place in a priſon, incloſed by high walls, it will continue to exert its baneful powers with various degrees of malignity, notwithſtanding all the cautions which may be employed to counteract its influence: and it is therefore recommended, as *eſſential* to ſalubrity, that a dry moat, with ſhelving ſides, like a line of circumvallation, ſhould ſurround, at a proper diſtance, the place of confinement; that from the bottom of this moat a wall ſhould be raiſed, twenty-five feet in height; but that the top of it ſhould not exceed the level of the ſoil. I apprehend that this mode of incloſure is impracticable in large towns, where an extent of land adequate to it, with a proper drainage, can ſeldom be obtained; that it would diminiſh the terrors of impriſonment to the ſpectators without, and to the malefactors within; that it might afford means of dangerous communication between them; that it is in no ſituation indiſpenſably neceſſary; and that the forcible manner in which it is urged, by ſuch reſpectable authority, may render

render the viſitation of moſt gaols, on their preſent unalterable conſtruction, too alarming to be undertaken by any honorary inſpectors, whether delegated in rotation from the magiſtracy, as Mr. Howard recommends, or appointed by authority of parliament. I ſhall not treſpaſs either on your time or my own, by engaging in the diſcuſſion of each of theſe topics: But I feel it incumbent on me to ſubmit, to your candid conſideration, the reaſons which lead me to controvert the opinion, "that walls above the level "of the inhabited ſurface are incompatible with "the neceſſary ventilation of a priſon."

EVER ſince the receipt of your letter, I have paid particular attention to the action of the wind in the court-yard at the back of my dwelling houſe, which is a quadrangular area of about three thouſand two hundred and forty ſquare feet, in the center of which are planted a few trees and ſhrubs. On the north ſide it is ſcreened by the houſe, which is three ſtories high, and eighteen yards in length. The ſouth ſide is occupied by a ſtable, coach-houſe, &c. On each of the other ſides, lower offices are erected; but behind theſe, conſiderable buildings riſe, the property of my neighbours. This area, therefore, is as much ſecluded from ventilation as the court-yards in many of our priſons; yet I have uniformly obſerved, that a very gentle wind ſuffices to give motion to the ſhrubs, and even

even to blow about the ſtraw and other light bodies on the flagged pavement, with which it is environed. The ſun-ſhine alſo, on the calmeſt day, cannot fail, by the heat which it communicates, to diſſipate the noxious vapours, and renovate the air. And every ſhower of rain performs the ſame ſalutary office.

THE means of obviating contagion, or the antidotes to it where it ſubſiſts, ſeem to be threefold. 1. Such as weaken its energy by *dilution*, or by a minute diviſion of its particles. 2. Such as operate ſolely on the human body, by counteracting its ſuſceptibility of infection. 3. Such as affect the poiſon itſelf, rendering it innoxious, by producing ſome chemical or other change in its nature. A familiar analogy may, at once, illuſtrate and confirm this propoſition. It is well known, that a grain of tartar emetic will excite vomiting. But if this antimonial preparation be diſſolved in a very large portion of water, the emetic power, which it poſſeſſed, will be deſtroyed. The ſame loſs of power will enſue, if a doſe of opium be adminiſtered, either previouſly or in conjunction with it, by which the ſtomach will become inſenſible to its action. And, laſtly, if an alkaline ſalt be added to it, the decompoſition thus produced will render it inert. A knowledge of theſe ſeveral correctives of contagion is intereſting to the magiſtrate as well as to the phyſician. But the moſt important of them, and what is now chiefly to be conſidered, is *dilution*, which may, I truſt, be accompliſhed, ſo as to obviate the communication of infection, by ſmaller ſupplies of freſh air, than you ſeem to apprehend.

CONTAGION, like all other poiſons, muſt ſubſiſt in ſome definite quantity, or degree of concentration, to be capable of producing its deleterious effects. And though the *minimum*, or leaſt point of activity, under which, when reduced by diffuſion, it becomes innoxious, hath not, and perhaps cannot, be preciſely aſcertained, yet we have ſufficient evidence to ſatisfy us, that this ſubſiſts at no great diſtance from its ſource. Dr. Mackenzie, who practiſed phyſic thirty years in the cities of Smyrna and Conſtantinople, aſſures us, that he was never afraid to go into a large houſe wherein a perſon lay under the plague, provided the patient was confined to one room. And the Rev. Thomas Dawes, chaplain to the Britiſh factory at Aleppo, in his account of a dreadful peſtilence which raged with ſuch violence in that place, in the years 1761 and 1762, that from two to three hundred perſons were buried daily, relates, that the plague twice broke out in two houſes adjoining to that in which the Britiſh Conſul lived: But although, according to the cuſtom of the eaſt, they conſtantly ſlept, during the months of July and Auguſt, in the open

open air on the houſe top, and a Franciſcan friar, whoſe bed was only ſix yards diſtant from that of Mr. Dawes (both being placed near a wall eight feet high, by which the terraces of the two houſes were ſeparated), died of the diſeaſe after two days illneſs, yet he and all the family eſcaped infection. I ſhall recite a more remarkable fact from the authority of my late honoured friend, Sir John Pringle, which ſtill further illuſtrates what has been advanced. In the year 1750, on the ſeventh of May, the ſeſſions commenced at the Old Baily, and continued ſeveral days, during which time more criminals were tried; and a greater multitude was preſent, than uſual. This court is only thirty feet ſquare; and the corruption of the air was aggravated by the foul ſteams of the bail-dock, and of two rooms opening into it, in which the priſoners were the whole day crowded together, till they were brought forth to take their trial. The bench conſiſted of ſix perſons, four of whom died of the gaol-diſtemper, together with two or three of the council, one of the under ſheriffs, ſeveral of the Middleſex jury, and above forty other perſons. It is to be noted, that the Chief Juſtice, who ſat on the Lord Mayor's right-hand, eſcaped; whilſt his Lordſhip, with the reſt of the bench on his left, was ſeized with the infection; that the Middleſex jury, on the ſame ſide of the court,

 loſt

loſt many, whilſt the London jury, oppoſite to them, received no injury; and that, of the multitude preſent, but one or two, or at moſt a ſmall number, of thoſe that were on the ſide of the court to the Lord Mayor's right-hand, were taken ill. Sir John Pringle aſcribes this partial action of contagion to the opening of a window at the end of the court moſt diſtant from the bench, by which he deems it probable that the poiſonous miaſms were directed to, and accumulated in, that part of the hall where the fatality ſo remarkably occurred. And I think we are equally warranted to conclude, from his narrative, that the air of the whole court, muſt have been contaminated, and that a moderate degree of dilution ſufficed to render the contagious particles innoxious.

Thus far I had written more than a month ago, as you will perceive by the date of my letter. Succeſſive and very urgent engagements have diſſipated my thoughts on this intereſting ſubject, and ſtill continue to engroſs my time. I hope you will not infer from the obſervations, which I have with much freedom ſuggeſted to you, that I regard the ventilation of gaols as an object of little importance; for it appears to me to claim the moſt ſerious attention, ſo far as it can be rendered compatible with the eſſential purpoſes of confinement. And, I rejoice to find, that

that Mr. Blackburne, an ingenious architect now employed in this county, and in various other parts of England, in the erection of new prisons, proposes to surround them with a wall of no great height, but covered at the top with *chevaux de frise*, which will afford perfect security, at the same time that it is pervious to the wind.

I MEANT to have offered to you some hints concerning the accommodation, clothing, diet, indulgences, and medical treatment of the prisoners, as they relate to the prevention or cure of the gaol-distemper. But I have at present no leisure to digest my thoughts; and it is probable they would convey little information to one who has so fully considered these subjects. When you see Dr. Jebb, be pleased to present my best respects to him: He has a claim to the warm esteem of every lover of his country.

THIS letter will be conveyed to you by Mr. Blackburne. I am called to a meeting of our magistrates, which is to be held to-day for the purpose of conferring with him on the erection of a new prison here.

I HAVE the honour to be, with very cordial respect,

SIR,

Your most faithful humble servant,

T. P.

REMARKS

RELATIVE TO THE IMPROVEMENT OF THE

MANCHESTER INFIRMARY;

COMMUNICATED TO THE

EDITOR of the GENTLEMAN'S MAGAZINE (a).

MANCHESTER, MARCH 19.

IN confequence of Mr. Howard's vifit, the beginning of laft year, to the infirmary at Manchefter, and of the remarks which he communicated concerning the general ftate of it, the following refolution was voted by the weekly board of truftees on the eighteenth of February, 1788:

" ORDERED, that all the phyficians, furgeons, " and vifiting apothecaries, and fuch other per- " fons as they fhall think proper to affift them, " be requefted to examine into the ftate of all the " wards, with refpect to their ventilation, and to " the cleanlinefs and condition of the beds and " furniture; and to report their opinion of the

(a) Inferted in the Gent. Mag. for March 1789, p. 191.

" fame

" ſame, in writing, to the next quarterly board; " and to meet for that purpoſe in the infirmary, " every Thurſday, at eleven o'clock until they have " given in their report."

THIS *reſolution* induced me to offer the following REMARKS to my brethren of the faculty, previous to the formation of our report. And as they may be applicable to other infirmaries, perhaps you will give them a place in your valuable miſcellany. The peruſal of Mr. Howard's excellent work *on Lazarettos*, of which he has lately favoured me with a copy, has renewed my attention to the POLITY of HOSPITALS. You may, therefore, expect a further correſpondence on this very intereſting topic, if the preſent hints meet with a favourable reception from your readers.

REMARKS *relative to the* IMPROVEMENT *of the* MANCHESTER INFIRMARY.

MARCH 10, 1788.

VENTILATION, cleanlineſs, and the numbers, ſtate, and accommodation of the patients, are the chief cauſes which affect the ſalubrity of the air in hoſpitals. And I ſhall take the liberty of offering a few remarks on each, as referable to the infirmary at Mancheſter.

 1. *Ventilation.*

1. *Ventilation.* Adequate ſupplies of *freſh* air are eſſential to its *purity:* But the *temperature* of it muſt alſo be regarded, with a view to *ſalubrity.* For cold is not only ungrateful to the feelings of the ſick, commonly very acute, but, in many diſeaſes, is injurious by its ſedative action; and has often been ſuſpected of giving energy to infection. The ventilation too ſhould be accompliſhed without any current of wind, perceptible at leaſt by the patients; for, ignorant of the nature and effects of contagion, they have no apprehenſions of danger from it, but have ſtrong prejudices againſt a flow of cool air, eſpecially when in bed or aſleep. Theſe prejudices, if they are to be deemed ſuch, claim not only tenderneſs, but indulgence: For, though ſilenced by authority, they will operate ſecretly and forcibly on the mind, by creating fear, anxiety, and watchfulneſs.

The grates, in the large wards of the infirmary, appear to be of inſufficient dimenſions to produce a due degree of warmth to the patients who are at a conſiderable diſtance from the fire. Yet, to ſuch who are near it, the heat is at preſent, perhaps, incommodious and unwholeſome. A frame of wood, lined with tin, like a kitchen haſter, ſhould therefore be placed on each ſide of the chimney, which would reflect warmth on the patients remote from, and be a defence to thoſe who

who are contiguous to it. The draught through the chimney would alſo be thus greatly increaſed, and the air of the chamber rendered more ſalubrious, both with reſpect to purity and temperature.

NEAR the fire there is a conſtant flow upwards of rarefied hot air, which is accumulated near the cieling. A ſupply of freſh air, therefore, from the outſide of the building, and from the galleries, might be conveyed to each ſide of the chimney, through pipes opening about two feet below the top of the room, by which the air would be warmed without contamination, and retain ſufficient ſpecific gravity to deſcend. Theſe pipes might be carried from the chimney, along the cieling, to its center, by which the warm and freſh air would be more equally diffuſed through the whole chamber.

ALL the ſaſhes ſhould be made to ſlide downwards, that, acccording to the ſeaſon of the year, more or leſs air may be admitted into the chambers of the ſick. Locks or bolts ſhould be contrived for the opening of the ſaſhes, that the nurſes or the patients may not have it in their power to cloſe them, when ſuch ventilation is deemed neceſſary. In cold weather, a thin board, of the length of the window, and ſloping upwards, ſhould be fixed at the top of the ſaſh frame, ſo as to direct the air which enters towards the cieling.

ing. A portion of each tranſom window, at the back of the infirmary, may be hung on a ſwivel, with the ſame precautions, as to its aperture, which have been recommended for the ſaſhes. The admiſſion of air by openings in the architraves of the doors, or in the doors themſelves, is an improvement adopted in ſeveral of the wards, and ſhould be extended to all of them. And, as their ſupplies of air muſt be derived from the galleries of the hoſpital, care ſhould be taken that they are perfectly well ventilated.

In the ſummer ſeaſon, when fires are laid aſide, the uſe of Dr. Hales's ventilator, in the way recommended by Sir John Pringle, would be adviſable.—" By them," ſays he, " we might " hope for a thorough purification of the air in " every ward; and working them might be a " good exerciſe for the convaleſcents."

2. *Cleanlineſs.* The matron of the houſe ſhould be ſtrictly enjoined to attend to the frequent renewal and airing of the bed-clothes, and to the waſhing of the blankets, quilts, &c. ſince theſe, being of a ſoft and porous texture, are diſpoſed to imbibe and to retain putrid and contagious effluvia.

Scouring the chamber floors at ſeaſonable times is indiſpenſably neceſſary. Yet, as the damp exhalations they occaſion may, in ſome caſes, be injurious, hot water with tolerably pure ſoap lyes ſhould

ſhould be employed to expedite the operation, to render it more complete, and to diminiſh the generation of cold.

Dry-rubbing, *with ſand*, is a practice which ſhould be forbidden. It fouls the furniture, diſtracts the patients with noiſe, offends the lungs by the duſt it raiſes, and may give diſperſion and activity to many morbific particles.

All the wards and the galleries ſhould be white-waſhed with hot lime annually, and oftener when malignant diſtempers have prevailed. The frame work of the beds ſhould, at the ſame time, be well ſcoured. It would be an expence alſo, fully compenſated by its benefits, if the flock-beds were on ſuch occaſions removed.

3. *The number, ſtate, and accommodation of the patients.* The contamination of the air ariſes chiefly from the crowding too many ſick perſons together in one chamber. Sir John Pringle lays it down as a rule, in the eſtabliſhment of military hoſpitals, "to admit ſo few invalids into each "ward, that a perſon, unacquainted with the "danger of bad air, might imagine there was "room to take in double or triple the number." If the dimenſions of our infirmary, and the preſſing claims for admiſſion into it, be inſurmountable obſtacles to the adoption of this rule, permit me, however, to ſuggeſt the propriety of making a diviſion in all the larger wards. Additional

tional ſides would thus be formed, which would afford a more favourable poſition for the beds, by ſeparating them from each other. Ventilation would be increaſed by the conſtruction of new fire-places, &c. and the temperature of the air would be rendered much more equal, comfortable, and ſalubrious. This improvement would alſo tend to obviate the ſpread of contagion, and would greatly diminiſh the injury, which the patients muſt ſuſtain from the multiplied ſpectacles of ſuffering, to which they are now witneſſes.

SINCE theſe obſervations were written, I have ſeen and examined the new patent-furnaces, called Imperial Stoves. They appear to be well adapted to give both warmth and ventilation to large rooms, and might be uſed with advantage in the infirmary. By an ingenious improvement in their conſtruction, the air is heated in an earthen, not in a metallic tube, by which its ſalubrity remains perfectly unimpaired. The price of theſe ſtoves is from three to ten guineas, and is proportionate to their ſize and elegance of form.

FINIS.

INDEX.

A.

ANIMALS,

INDEX.

B.

D.

F.

G.

HÆMOPTYSIS,

H.

I.

J.

L.

M.

N.

I N D E X.

O.

P.

Pomponius

Q.

R.

INDEX.

T.

V.

I N D E X.

W.

Y.

Z.

N. B. In the Errata, line penult. for *tracþæa* read *trachea*.

THE END.

Printed in the United States
By Bookmasters